To Dr. William P. Sears,

Kindest regards
and best wishes.

Louis A. Perkiel

J. K. Lane

MEDICAL TERMINOLOGY
SIMPLIFIED

MEDICAL TERMINOLOGY
SIMPLIFIED

by

LOUIS L. PERKEL, B.S., M.D., F.A.C.P.

Diplomate, American Board of Internal Medicine and
Sub-specialty, Gastroenterology
Professor of Gastroenterology, Seton Hall College of Medicine
Jersey City, New Jersey
Director, Department of Gastroenterology and
The Intern and Resident Training Program
Jersey City Medical Center

Foreword by

CHARLES L. BROWN, M.D., F.A.C.P.

Dean, Seton Hall College of Medicine
Jersey City, New Jersey

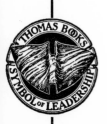

CHARLES C THOMAS · PUBLISHER
Springfield · Illinois · U.S.A.

CHARLES C THOMAS • PUBLISHER

BANNERSTONE HOUSE

301-327 East Lawrence Avenue, Springfield, Illinois, U.S.A.

Published simultaneously in the British Commonwealth of Nations by

BLACKWELL SCIENTIFIC PUBLICATIONS, LTD., OXFORD, ENGLAND

Published simultaneously in Canada by

THE RYERSON PRESS, TORONTO

Copyright 1958, by CHARLES C THOMAS • PUBLISHER

Library of Congress Catalog Card Number: 58-8431

With THOMAS BOOKS careful attention is given to all details of manu-
facturing and design. It is the Publisher's desire to present books that are
satisfactory as to their physical qualities and artistic possibilities and appropriate for their particular use. THOMAS BOOKS will be true to those laws of
quality that assure a good name and good will.

Printed in the United States of America

TO
FLORA

FOREWORD

Words, being sounds having a meaning, and the writing or printing representing such sounds, are implements by which we communicate our thoughts. Effectively assembled, words form a language which, written or spoken, becomes an art only perfected by constant and meticulous practice. The art and the skill in the use and choice of words is most pertinent in the clarity of expression in the field of medicine. The combination and arrangement of words, that is phrases, are capable of expressing thoughts in a particular way and effectiveness. All too often the medical profession falls heir to the use of a kind of jargon in every day communication, both in speech and writing, which seems confusing and meaningless except to the members of the profession itself.

In the education period, as well as in the practice of medicine, no more fitting comment could be made than that of Peter Roget in the introduction in his *International Thesaurus* (Thomas Y. Crowell Company, New York): "It is of the utmost consequence that strict accuracy should regulate our use of language, and that every one should acquire the power and the habit of expressing his thoughts with perspicuity and correctness."

With changing concepts of the nature of many diseases and the rapid expansion of knowledge, the tremendous increase in the vocabulary in medicine has been inevitable and increasingly complicated. The specific meaning of new terms has posed a great responsibility on the medical educator and writer.

In this small volume Doctor Perkel, as a result of his long experience in teaching young physicians, nurses, and other personnel in the hospital staff, has captured a way of making the significance and use of common medical terms and phraseology both entertaining and meaningful.

The style and arrangement are fascinating. Start to look for a word and you find you keep on looking for more and more words. Pick up the little book for browsing and you will not want to lay it down until you have finished it.

CHARLES L. BROWN, M.D.

PREFACE

Understanding medical terminology is essential for medical, dental and nursing students; medical secretaries, librarians, technicians and other affiliates of the medical sciences. Just as a skilled craftsman is familiar with and knows how to use the *tools* of his trade, so members of the medical or allied professions, or any of their auxiliaries, should understand and know how to properly use the *tools* of the profession, namely, MEDICAL TERMS.

Speaking English correctly is a sign of an educated person. By the same token, being well versed in medical terminology is a sign of an educated professional person, be he physician, dentist, nurse, secretary, or technician. Besides, understanding medical terms and knowing how to use them properly is necessary in exchanging ideas, teaching and research, all recognized as activities essential for progress in the medical sciences.

For more than twenty-five years the author has been lecturing on this subject to student nurses, medical secretaries and other medical ancillaries at the Jersey City Medical Center. The first year students of the Seton Hall College of Medicine and Dentistry, recently established at the Jersey City Medical Center, are also receiving these lectures.

This book is the result of the expansion and elaboration of the notes and outlines used in these courses, aided by the accumulated experience gained from the latter. It is hoped that it will serve as a useful and

practical guide to the important subject of MEDICAL
TERMINOLOGY, heretofore relatively neglected in the
curricula of most schools.

Although this volume contains considerable factual
medical information, it is not, in the slightest degree,
intended to serve as a course in medicine, abridged or
otherwise. The informative data necessarily presented
herein is specifically for the purpose of illustrating the
methods of learning how to understand medical terminology and correcting prevalent misuse of medical
terms.

If, perchance, in the use of this book, the reader does
acquire new knowledge, he will surely benefit profes-
sionally thereby, which, after all, is the author's goal.

The study of medical terminology is not only educational but is also fascinating, especially to those in
the medical profession and allied fields. In searching
for and analyzing the origins of many terms in and out
of current usage, one comes across engrossing bits of
colorful data concerning mythology and the history of
medicine. Besides, many ancient myths, as well as
truths, about the human body, health and disease are
uncovered. A liberal sampling of this interesting information will be presented in the pages that follow.

The author gratefully acknowledges his indebtedness
to his wife, Flora Perkel, R.N., for her invaluable help,
both physically and spiritually, in the preparation of
the manuscript. Without her encouragement, advice
and constructive criticism, this book could not have
been written.

Jersey City, New Jersey

LOUIS L. PERKEL, M.D.

CONTENTS

MEDICAL TERMINOLOGY
SIMPLIFIED

INTRODUCTION

M EDICINE, BEING a systematic science, must have as its *language* an accurate and never-changing vocabulary. Medical terms must be so precise that there can be no chance of misunderstanding or misinterpretation of their meanings. It is therefore understandable that medical scientists, both ancient and modern, have resorted to the so-called dead or *classic* languages for descriptive terms. The definitions of these terms, in contrast to those of words of modern languages, are exact and changeless through the ages and throughout most of the world. Centuries of experience support this statement.

Constant advances in medical science require the frequent coining of new medical terms such as the names of new conditions, diseases, tests, signs, symptoms, drugs and other methods of treatment. Here, again, for the reasons just stated, recourse is made to the classic languages for the most appropriate, descriptive and accurate components of the new terms.

Hence, medical terms are derived mostly from the Greek and Latin. The writings of the Greek physician, Hippocrates (460-370 B.C.), considered the Father of Medicine, furnish us with the first organized collection of medical words, most of which are in present use. His famous, scholarly document, the OATH OF HIPPO-CRATES, though written more than 2000 years ago, is still timely and persists as the ethical code of the profession, sworn to by every physician on his day of grad-

3

uation from medical school.

After the decline of the Greek era many Greek words were latinized by the then influential Romans. Most prominent of these was the Roman physician, Galen (131-201 A.D.), whose father was Greek. He assiduously followed the teachings of Hippocrates and his writings constituted medical authority for more than 1500 years. He also handed down a long list of natural (vegetable) pharmaceutical preparations known as "galenicals."

Latin has been the universal language of science and medicine for many centuries, yet, within its framework, many Greek words persist either in their original form or recognizably latinized. The Romans added these Greek words to their own Latin in the make-up of their medical terminology. This accounts for the bilingual (Greek and Latin) roots from which many present medical terms are derived.

Those who are concerned over their failure to have studied the classic languages can be assured that knowledge of Greek and Latin, though helpful, is not essential in learning medical terminology.

Besides GREEK and LATIN, other sources of medical terms and some of their contributions are: the ANGLO-SAXON, *arm, ear, elbow, ache, head, breast, bone, boil, retch, crutch, gall, gut, hip, rib,* etc.; the FRENCH, *tic, caffein, bougie, contracoup, bruit, accoucheur, truss, ballottement, tissue, debridement, tourniquet, grand mal, petit mal, trocar, rale, malady, grippe,* etc.; the ITALIAN, *malaria, quarantine, belladonna, influenza, douche* (from doccia), *pellagra, scarlatina* (from scarlotto), etc.; the GERMAN, *anlage, magenstrasse* and *mittelschmerz;* the ARABIC, chiefly chemical names as *syrup, elixir, aniline, tartar, senna, alcohol, alkali, sugar,* and the anatomical term *nucha* (the nape of the neck); and a sprinkling of others of miscellaneous origin. The total number of these terms from other sources is so small as to be insignificant compared to the overwhelming majority of those of Greek and Latin origin.

Webster's dictionary defines ETYMOLOGY as: "the study of the origin or derivation of a word as shown by its analysis into elements, by pointing out the root or primitive upon which it is based, or by referring to an earlier form in its parent language." Inasmuch as MEDICAL ETYMOLOGY is actually the basis of MEDICAL TERMINOLOGY, the principles stated in the above definition will be followed literally in the unfolding of the theme of this book.

PRINCIPLES OF WORD
CONSTRUCTION

M EDICAL TERMS, as is true with ordinary English words, are made up of *roots* alone, in combination with *prefixes,* or *suffixes,* or both. In certain words *combining terms* are used in place of suffixes.

To acquire a medical vocabulary one must first memorize the important roots, prefixes and suffixes. Then one should make it a practice to analyze each medical term encountered, breaking it down to its component elements. For example, the term GASTRO-ENTERITIS is a combination of GASTR(O), meaning *stomach;* ENTER, meaning *intestines;* and -ITIS, meaning *inflammation of.* The definition of the term is readily recognized as *inflammation of the stomach and intestines.* Similarly, the term OSTEOCHONDROMA is broken down to OSTE(O), meaning *bone;* CHONDR, meaning *cartilage;* and -OMA, meaning *tumor of;* all adding up to *tumor of bone and cartilage.*

The term NEPHROLITHIASIS is made up of NEPHR-(O), meaning *kidney;* LITH, meaning *stone;* and -(I)ASIS, meaning *condition of being;* the whole term meaning *condition of kidney stone(s).* Even a more lengthy, complex and, at first glance, unintelligible term, as OTORHINOLARYNGOLOGY, loses its terror and becomes simple when one recognizes its component roots, as OT(O), *ear;* RHIN(O), *nose;* LARYNG(O), *throat;* and the combining term, -LOGY; *study of.* By

7

simply adding these together, the meaning of the term becomes obvious, namely, *the study of (diseases of) the ear, nose and throat.*

A longer, and perhaps even more foreboding, term as CHOLECYSTOELECTROCOAGULECTOMY is easily analyzed by breaking it down to: CHOLE, *gall;* CYST, *bladder;* ELECTROCOAGUL, *electrocoagulation;* and -ECTOMY, *removal of;* all adding up to *extirpation (removal) of the gall bladder by electrocoagulation.*

Proficiency in understanding medical terminology is attained by constant *word analysis,* as described and exemplified above, supplemented by reference to a good *medical dictionary* for the *derivation, analysis of the component elements* and *definition* of each newly encountered medical term.

Conversely, a medical term is constructed by combining a *prefix* or *suffix,* or both, with a *root.* Frequently, several roots are *joined* to form a term, as in CARDIOVASCULAR, CEREBROSPINAL, and NEUROPSYCHIATRY. The same root may appear in many terms combined with various prefixes, suffixes or other roots. For example, the root UR(O) or UR(IA), meaning *urine,* is combined with the prefix AN-, meaning *absence of,* to form the term ANURIA; with the prefix DYS-, meaning *painful* or *difficult,* to form the term DYSURIA; with the root HEMA(T), meaning *blood,* to form the term HEMATURIA; with the root GLYCO(S), meaning *sugar,* to form the term GLYCOSURIA; with the root PY, meaning *pus,* to form the term PYURIA; with the combining term -LOGY, meaning *study of,* to form the term UROLOGY; with the combining term -GRAM, meaning *record,* to form the term UROGRAM: with the root BIL(IN), meaning *bile,* to form the term UROBILIN; etc. Similarly, the root CARD(IUM) or CARD(IA), meaning

heart, may be combined with ENDO- to form ENDOCARD-
IUM; with MYO- to form MYOCARDIUM; with PERI- to
form PERICARDIUM; with BRADY- to form BRADYCARDIA;
with TACHY- to form TACHYCARDIA; with PERI- and
-ITIS to form PERICARDITIS; with -LOGY to form CARDIO-
LOGY; etc.

As in English, a prefix can be used with various
roots to form words of different meanings. For example, the prefix DYS-, meaning *painful* or *difficult,* is
found in such terms as DYSPNEA, *difficult breathing;*
DYSMENORRHEA, *painful menstruation;* DYSPHAGIA,
difficult swallowing; etc. The Greek alpha privative,
A- or AN-, is a commonly used prefix meaning *without,
absence of,* or *lack of.* Examples are ANACIDITY, AN-
OREXIA, ANESTHESIA, AVASCULAR, APNEA, ANEMIA, etc.

Frequently used suffixes are -ITIS, -OMA, -ASIS or
-OSIS, -OTOMY, -OSTOMY, and -ECTOMY. -ITIS is found
in numerous terms, such as APPENDICITIS, GASTRITIS,
TONSILLITIS, COLITIS, etc., indicating *inflammation of*
the particular organ to whose name it is added. -OMA
means *tumor of;* (OSTEOMA, SARCOMA, CARCINOMA,
HEMANGIOMA). -ASIS or -OSIS means *condition of being;*
(DIVERTICULOSIS, NEUROSIS, HYPOCHRONDRIASIS).
-OTOMY means *cutting into;* (GASTROTOMY). -OSTOMY
means *making a mouth* or *opening into;* (GASTRO-
STOMY). -ECTOMY means *excision of;* (GASTRECTO-
MY).

In both Greek and Latin words, the combining form
of the root is usually in the genitive case which may be
quite different from the nominative. For instance, the
nominative of the Greek word for *tooth* is ODOUS but
it is from ODONTOS, the genitive, that the combining
form ODONT is derived. Similarly, the Latin word for
tooth is DENS but it is DENTIS, the genitive, from which

the combining form DENT is derived.

In certain compound terms where the second component begins with a consonant, the vowel "o" is placed between the two components for the sake of euphony. Examples are NEUR(O)LOGY, CEREBR(O)-SPINAL, ARTERI(O)SCLEROSIS, DERM(O)GRAPHIA, TEST(O)STERONE, etc.

If in the joining of two components of a term two vowels come together, then, again for euphony, the first vowel is dropped. Examples are: PARA-ENTERAL becomes PARENTERAL; HYPO-ALGESIA becomes HYPAL-GESIA and META-HEMOGLOBIN becomes METHEMO-GLOBIN; PARA-OTID becomes PAROTID; DIA-URETIC becomes DIURETIC; etc.

In certain terms the consonant ending the prefix is changed to that which begins the root that follows:, e.g., SUB-PURATION becomes SUPPURATION; EX-FERENT becomes EFFERENT; SUB-POSITORY becomes SUPPOSI-TORY; EX-FUSION becomes EFFUSION; IN-MERSION becomes IMMERSION; etc.

In certain words, the addition of a prefix may change the vowel of the root it modifies; thus OB-CAPUT becomes OCCIPUT; BI-CAPUT becomes BICEPS; IN-IACTUS becomes INJECT; etc.

COMMON ROOTS OR STEMS

A̶LL ROOTS listed are derived from the Greek, except those in brackets and followed by the letter "L", indicating their Latin origin. Each root, shown by its combining form, is followed by its definition and examples of terms containing it. The same applies to the lists of prefixes and suffixes that follow:

ACR(O) . . . . .extremity,
                   end or
                   point . . . . . (ACROMEGALY)
                                (ACROCEPHALY)

ADEN(O);
  [GLANS,
  GLAND(ULA)-L] . . gland . . . . . (ADENITIS)
                               (GLANDULAR)

ANGI(O);
  [VAS(O),
  VASCULAR-L] . . . . .vessel . . . . . (ANGIOMA)
                               (VASCULARITY)

ARTHR(O) . . . . .joint . . . . . . (ARTHRITIS)
                               (ARTHROPATHY)

BIO, -OBE . . . . life . . . . (BIOLOGY)
                               (MICROBE)

BLEPHAR(ON);
  [PALPEBRA-L] . . . .eyelid . . . . . (BLEPHARITIS)
                               (PALPEBRAL)

BOL . . . . .building or
                   throwing . . (CATABOLISM)
                               (ANABOLIC)

CEPHAL(O);
  [CAPUT,
  CAPIT(IS)-L].... .head...... (CEPHALIC)
                           (DECAPITATE)

CARDI(O);
  [COR,
  CORD(IS)-L]..... heart..... (CARDIAC)
                           (PRECORDIAL)

CELI(O),
  COELI(O)....... belly or
                abdomen.. (CELIOTOMY)
                           (CELIORRHAPHY)

CHEIL(O);
  [LABI(UM)-L]... .lip....... (CHEILITIS)
                           (LABIAL)

CHIR(O);
  [MAN(US)-L].... hand..... (CHIROPODY)
                           (MANUAL)

CHOL(E)(O);
  [BIL(I)-L]....... bile...... (CHOLECY-
                           STECTOMY)
                           (BILIARY)

CHONDR(O);
  [CARTILAG(O)-L]. cartilage... (CHONDROMA)
                           (SYNCHONDROSIS)

CLYSIS........... .drenching. .(HYPODERMOCLYSIS)
                           (VENOCLYSIS)

[CORTEX,
  CORTIC(ES)-L]... bark, or
               outside
               layer of
               an organ.. (ADRENAL CORTEX)
                           (CORTICOSTERONE)

[COST(O)-L]....... rib....... (INTERCOSTAL)
                           (COSTOVERTEBRAL)

CRAN(I)..........skull......(CRANIOTOMY)
                            (CRANIUM)
CYAN(O).........,blue......(CYANOSIS)
                            (ACROCYANOSIS)
CYST;
  [VESIC(O)-L].... bladder... (CYSTITIS)
                            (VESICAL)
CYT(E);
  [CELL(A)-L].....cell......(CYTOPLASM) ·
                            (AGRANULOCYTE)
DACTYL(O);
  [DIGIT(US)-L]....finger.....(DACTYLITIS)
                            (DIGITAL)
DACRY(O);
  [LACHRYM(A)-L]. tear...... (DACRYOCYSTITIS)
                            (LACHRYMAL)
DERM(A)(AT)(O);
  [CUT(IS)-L]..... skin...... (DERMATOLOGY)
                            (CUTICLE)
DIPS(O).......... drink..... (DIPSOMANIAC)
                            (POLYDIPSIA)
[DORS(I)(O)-L].... back or
                  posterior.. (DORSUM)
                            (DORSIFLEXION)
EMET, EMESIS;
  [VOM(ERE)-L]... vomit.....(HYPEREMESIS)
                            (VOMITUS)
ENCEPHAL(O);
  [CEREBR(UM)-L]. brain..... (ENCEPHALOGRAM)
                            (CEREBRAL)
ENTER(O);
  [INTESTIN(US)-L].intestine...(ENTERITIS)
                            (INTESTINAL)
ERYTHR(O);
  [RUB(ER)-L].....red.......(ERYTHROCYTE)

(RUBEFACIENT)
ESTHESI(O) . . . . feeling. . . . (ESTHESIOMETER)
(PARESTHESIA)
[EXCIS(IO)-L]. . . . . . to cut out. . (EXCISE)
(EXCISION)
[FEBRI-L]. . . . . fever. . . . . (FEBRILE)
(FEBRIFACIENT)
GALACT(O);
  [LACT(O)-L]. . . . .milk. . . . . .(GALACTAGOGUE)
(LACTATE)
GASTR(O);
  [STOMACH(US)-L] .stomach. . .(GASTRITIS)
(STOMACHIC)
GEN(E). . . . . .producing,
           family,
           race or
           origin. . . . .(GENETICS)
(PATHOGEN)
[GENUS,
  GENER(A)-L]. . . . race, kind
           or group. . .(GENERIC)
(GENUS)
GER(AS)(ON),
  PRESBY. . . . . . . .aged. . . . . .(GERIATRICS)
(PRESBYOPIA)
GLOSS(A);
  [LINGU(A)-L]. . . .tongue. . . . (GLOSSITIS)
(SUBLINGUAL)
GNOSIS. . . . . .knowledge. (DIAGNOSIS)
(PROGNOSIS)
GON(E), SPERM(A) . seed. . . . . .(GONAD)
(SPERMATIC)
GYNEC. . . . . .woman. . . .(GYNECIC)
(GYNECOLOGY)
HEM(AT)(O),

EMIA;
[SANGU(IS)-L]... .blood..... (HEMIC)
(SANGUINEOUS)
HEPAR, HEPAT(O) .. liver...... (HEPATOMA)
(HEPATITIS)
HYDR(O)(AT);
[AQU(A)-L]......water..... (DEHYDRATION)
(AQUEOUS)
HYPN(O);
[SOMN(US)-L],
[SOPOR-L]........sleep..... .(HYPNOSIS)
(INSOMNIA)
(SOPORIFIC)
HYSTER(O),
METR(A);
[UTER(US)-L]....womb..... .(HYSTERECTOMY)
(ENDOMETRITIS)
(UTERINE)
[INCIS(IO)-L]...... to cut
(into).... (INCISION)
(INCISURE)
LIP(O), STEAT(O);
[ADIPIS-L].......fat....... (LIPOMA)
(STEATORRHEA)
(ADIPOSE)
LITH(O).........stone..... (LITHIASIS)
(PHLEBOLITH)
LUMB(O)........loin...... (LUMBAR)
(LUMBAGO)
LYSIS........... .loosening
or a
breaking
down..... (DIALYSIS)
(HYDROLYSIS)
MAST(OS);

[MAMMA-L]......breast.....(MASTITIS)
                                          (MAMMARY)

[MEDULL(A)-L]....marrow or
central
part of an
organ.....(MEDULLA)
                                         (MEDULLOBLAST)

MELAN(O)........black.....(MELANOMA)
                                         (MELENA)

MEN(S)..........month....(MENSES)
                                         (DYSMENORRHEA)

METER...........measure...(THERMOMETER)
                                         (HYDROMETER)

MNES(IS).........memory...(AMNESIA)
                                         (ANAMNESIS)

MORPH(E)........form......(AMORPHOUS)
                                         (MORPHOLOGY)

MY(O);
   [MUSCUL(US)-L].muscle....(MYOMA)
                                         (MUSCULATURE)

MYEL(O)........marrow...(MYELITIS)
                                         (MYELOCYTE)

MYX(O)..........mucus....(MYXOMA)
                                         (MYXORRHEA)

NARC(O).........stupor....(NARCOTIC)
                                         (NARCOLEPSY)

NECR(O).........death.....(NECROPSY)
                                         (NECROSIS)

NEPHR(O); [REN-L].kidney....(NEPHRITIS)
                                         (RENAL)

NEUR(O).........nerve.....(NEURITIS)
                                         (NEUROLOGY)

NYCT(O); [NOCT-L].night.....(NYCTALOPIA)
                                         (NOCTURIA)

OMPHAL(O);

[UMBILIC(US)-L]. navel..... (OMPHALOTOMY)
                            (UMBILICAL)
OOPHOR(O);
  [OVARI(UM)-L]...ovary..... (OOPHORECTOMY)
                            (OVARIAN)
OPHTHALM(OS);
  [OCUL(US)-L]....eye.......(OPHTHALMOSCOPE)
                            (OCULIST)
ORCHI(D)(O);
  [TEST(IS)-L].....testicle....(ORCHITIS)
                            (TESTOTERONE)
OREX, ORECT......appetite...(HYPEROREXIA)
                            (ANORECTIC)
OSTE(O); [OS,
  OSS(IS)-L]......bone......(OSTEITIS)
                            (OSSEOUS)
OT(OS);
  [AUR(IS)-L]..... ear.......(OTITIS)
                            (AURICLE)
PATH(O).........disease....(PATHOLOGY)
                            (PSYCHOPATH)
PHAG(E)(O)......eat or
                  swallow...(BACTERIOPHAGE)
                            (PHAGOCYTE)
PHARMAC(O)......drug......(PHARMACY)
                            (PHARMACOLOGY)
PHAS(IA)........ speech....(APHASIA)
                            (PARAPHASIA)
PHLEB(O);
  [VEN(A)-L]......vein......(PHLEBITIS)
                            (VENOGRAPHY)
PHON(O); [VOX,
  VOC(IS)-L]......sound
                  or voice...(PHONETIC)
                            (VOCAL)

PHREN(O); [MENS,
   MENT(IS)-L].... .mind..... (PHRENOLOGY)
                                  (MENTAL)

PHYS(IS) .... .growth
                      (also
                      nature)... (EPIPHYSIS)
                                  (PHYSICS)

PLASIA, PLASM(A),
   PLAST......... .mold or
                    tissue
                    formation.. .(ANAPLASIA)
                              (NEOPLASM)
                              (PLASTIC)

PLEX, PLEG....... .stroke.... .(APOPLEXY)
                              (HEMIPLEGIA)

PNEA........... .breathing.. (DYSPNEA)
                              (HYPERPNEA)

PNEUM(A)(O)(AT) .breath
                    or air..... (PNEUMATOSIS)
                            (PNEUMOTHORAX)

PNEUMON(O);
   [PULMON-L]..... lung...... (PNEUMONITIS)
                              (PULMONIC)

POD(OS); [PES,
   PED(IS)-L]...... foot...... (PODIATRY)
                              (PEDAL)

PROCT(OS);
   [AN(US)-L]..... .anus or
                    rectum.... (PROCTITIS)
                              (ANAL)

PSYCH(O) .... .soul or
                    mind..... (PSYCHOLOGY)
                              (PSYCHOGENIC)

PY(O)........... .pus....... (PYEMIA)
                              (PYORRHEA)

PYEL(O) . . . . .pelvis of
                    kidney . . . . (PYELOGRAM)
                                   (PYELITIS)
RHIN(OS);
   [NAS(US)-L] . . . . . nose . . . . . . (RHINITIS)
                                   (NASAL)
SALPINX,
   SALPING(O) . . . . . fallopian
                    or uterine
                    tube . . . . . . (PYOSALPINX)
                                   (SALPINGITIS)
SARC(O), CREAS,
   CREAT(IN);
   [CARN(I)-L] . . . . . flesh . . . . . . (SARCOMA)
                                   (PANCREAS)
                                   (CARNIVEROUS)
SCLER(O) . . . . .hard . . . . . . (SCLEROSIS)
                                   (SCLERA)
SEPSIS, SEPTIC . . . . . putrefac-
                    tion, rot or
                    infection . . .(ASEPSIS)
                                   (SEPTICEMIA)
SIAL(O);
   [SALIV(A)-L] . . . . saliva . . . . . (SIALOLITH)
                                   (SALIVATION)
SIT(E) . . . . food . . . . . . (PARASITE)
                                   (SITOMANIA)
SOMA, SOMAT(OS);
   [CORP(US),
   CORPOR(IS)-L] . . . body . . . . . (SOMATIC)
                                   (CORPOREAL)
SPHYGM(O) . . . . pulse . . . . . (SPHYGMOMANO-
                                   METER)
                                   (SPHYGMOGRAPH)
SPLEN; [LIEN-L] . . . . spleen . . . . (SPLENIC)

(LIENITIS)

STETH(O);
　[PECTUS,
　PECTOR(IS)-L]... chest..... (STETHOSCOPE)
　　　　　　　　　　　　　　(PECTORAL)

STOM(A)(T);
　[OS, OR(IS)-L]... mouth.... (STOMATITIS)
　　　　　　　　　　　　　　(ORAL)

THELI(UM)....... nipple or
　　　　　　　　　layer of
　　　　　　　　　surface
　　　　　　　　　cells...... (EPITHELIOMA)
　　　　　　　　　　　　　　(ENDOTHELIUM)

THERM(O);
　[CALOR-L].......heat...... (THERMAL)
　　　　　　　　　　　　　　(CALORIMETER)

THROMB(O).......clot.......(THROMBUS)
　　　　　　　　　　　　　　(THROMBOCYTE)

TOX(I), TOXIC(O).. poison.... (TOXEMIA)
　　　　　　　　　　　　　　(TOXICOSIS)

TRACHEL(OS);
　[CERVIX,
　CERVIC(IS)-L]....neck......(TRACHELOTOMY)
　　　　　　　　　　　　　　(CERVICAL)

TRICH(O);
　[PIL(O)-L]...... hair...... (HYPERTRICHOSIS)
　　　　　　　　　　　　　　(PILONIDAL)

TROPH(Y)........nutrition...(ATROPHY)
　　　　　　　　　　　　　　(TROPHIC)

UR(IA), UR(O);
　[URIN(A)-L].....urine..... (ANURIA)
　　　　　　　　　　　　　　(UROGRAM)
　　　　　　　　　　　　　　(URINAL)

VARIX, VARIC(ES)...dilated
　　　　　　　　　vein...... (VARICECTOMY)

(VARICOSE)

[VENTRICUL(O)-L]..small
               cavity or
               pouch.....(VENTRICLE)
               (VENTRICULOGRAM)
[VENTR(O)-L].....anterior
               aspect of
               body or
               abdomen..(VENTRAL)
               (VENTROFIXATION)
[VERMI-L]........worm.....(VERMIFORM)
               (VERMIFUGE)
[VIT(A)-L].......life.......(VITAL)
               (DEVITALIZE)
ZOO(N)..........animal....(ZOOLOGY)
               (MICROZOON)
ZYM(O)..........ferment...(ENZYME)
               (ZYMASE)

SOME COMMON DENTAL ROOTS

[APEX, APIC(IS)-L].. tip or top..(APEX)
(APICAL)
ADAMANTIN(E).... very hard..(ADAMANTINOMA)
[CUSP-L]..........point or tip (BICUSPID)
(TRICUSPID)
[CLUS (from
CLAUDERE)-L]... to close... (MALOCCLUSION)
(OCCLUSAL)
[DENS, DENT(IS)-L]. tooth..... (DENTITION)
(DENTURE)
[CARIES-L]........ decay.....(CARIES)
(CARIOGENIC)
EPOULIS;
[GINGIV(A)-L]... gum......(EPULIS)
(GINGIVITIS)
GNATH(US)....... jaw.......(EUGNATHIC)
(DYSGNATHIC)
HALIT(US)........ breath.... (HALITOSIS)
ODONT(OS)....... tooth..... (ORTHODONTIA)
(ODONTOMA)
PROSTH(ES)(IS),
PROSTHETIC..... in addition.(PROSTHODONTIA)
(PROSTHETICS)
[PULP(A)-L]...... flesh......(PULPITIS)
(PULPOTOMY)

22

COMMON PREFIXES

A-, AN-. . . . . .without or
                        lack of. . . . (AGNOSIA)
                                     (ANEMIA)
AB-(L). . . . . away from.(ABORAL)
                                (ABNORMAL)
AD-(L). . . . . to, toward
                       or near to. .(ADRENAL)
                               (ADDUCTOR)
AMBI-(L). . . . . both. . . . . .(AMBIDEXTROUS)
                             (AMBIVALENT)
AMPH(I)(O)-. . . . . . both ways. (AMPHIBIOUS)
                             (AMPHOTERIC)
ANA-. . . . . up, again. . (ANATOMY)
                             (ANASTOMOSIS)
ANTE-(L). . . . . before. . . . (ANTERIOR)
                             (ANTECUBITAL)
ANTI-. . . . . .against. . . .(ANTISEPTIC)
                             (ANTIBIOTIC)
APO-. . . . . from or
                       away from.(APOPLEXY)
                             (APONEUROSIS)
AUTO-. . . . . self. . . . . .(AUTOLYSIS)
                             (AUTOPSY)
BI-, BIN-(L). . . . . . . two, twice
                       or double. .(BIMANUAL)
                             (BINAURAL)
                             (BIPED)
CATA-. . . . . down or
                       according

	to	(CATABOLISM)
		(CATARRH)
CIRCUM-(L)	around	(CIRCUMCISION)
		(CIRCUMOCULAR)
CO-, COM-, CON-(L) .	with	(CO-ENZYME)
		(COMMISSURE)
		(CONGENITAL)
CONTRA-(L)	against or opposite . . .	(CONTRALATERAL)
		(CONTRACOUP)
DE-(L)	away from .	(DEMENTIA)
		(DECIDUA)
DEXTRO-	right	(DEXTROCARDIA)
		(DEXTROMANUAL)
DIA-	through or across	(DIALYSIS)
		(DIAPHRAGM)
DIS-	apart from; negation . . .	(DISLOCATION)
		(DISINFECTION)
DI(S)-, DIPL(O)-	two, twice or double . .	(DIPLEGIA)
		(DIPLOPIA)
DYS-	difficult, painful or bad	(DYSPHAGIA)
		(DYSPNEA)
		(DYSPEPSIA)
E-, EC-,EX-(L)	out	(EVISCERATION)
		(ECCHYMOSIS)
		(EXPIRATION)
ECTO-	outside	(ECTODERM)
		(ECTOPLASM)
EM-, EN-	in	(EMPYEMA)
		(ENDEMIC)

ENDO-............within.... (ENDOCARDIUM)
                            (ENDOMETRIUM)
EPI-.............upon or on.(EPIDEMIC)
                            (EPIDERMIS)
EXTR(A)-(L)...... outside....(EXTRACELLULAR)
                            (EXTRINSIC)
EU-.............well...... (EUPHORIA)
                            (EUGENICS)
                            (EUTHYROID)
HEMI-............half...... (HEMIANOPSIA)
                            (HEMICRANIA)
HETERO-..........different
                 or other... (HETEROGENEOUS)
                            (HETEROPHILE)
HOMO-...........same..... (HOMOSEXUAL)
                            (HOMOGENEOUS)
HYPER-...........over,
                 above or
                 excessive.. (HYPERTENSION)
                            (HYPERPLASIA)
                            (HYPERTONIC)
HYPO-............under or
                 below.....(HYPODERMIC)
                            (HYPOTONIC)
IDIO-............peculiar to
                 itself......(IDIOPATHIC)
                            (IDIOVENTRICULAR)
IM-, IN-(L)........in (or not).(INJECTION)
                            (IMPERFORATE)
INFRA-(L).........below.....(INFRAORBITAL)
                            (INFRARED)
INTER-(L).........between... (INTERCOSTAL)
                            (INTERCELLULAR)
INTRA-(L).........within.... (INTRACUTANEOUS)
                            (INTRACELLULAR)

LEIO-. . . . . .smooth. . . .(LEIOMYOMA)
(LEIODERMIA)
LEUCO-; [ALB(A)-L]. white. . . . . (LEUCOPLAKIA)
(ALBINISM)
LEVO-(L). . . . . left. . . . . . .(LEVOROTATORY)
(LEVOGRAM)
MACRO-. . . . . .large. . . . . .(MACROCOCCUS)
(MACROCYTE)
MAL-. . . . . .bad. . . . . .(MALUNION)
(MALFORMATION)
MEGA-, MEGALO-. . . .great. . . . . (MEGACOLON)
(MEGALOCYTE)
MES(O)-;
[MEDI(O)-L]. . . . .middle. . . .(MESODERM)
(MEDIAL)
META-. . . . . .change,
after or
beyond. . . .(METASTASIS)
(METABOLISM)
MICRO-. . . . . small. . . . . (MICROCYTE)
(MICROSCOPE)
NEO-. . . . . .new. . . . . . (NEOPLASM)
(NEONATAL)
ORTHO-. . . . . right,
straight,
true or
upright. . . .(ORTHOPNEA)
(ORTHOSTATIC)
(ORTHOTONIC)
PAN-. . . . . all or
universal. . (PANDEMIC)
(PANHYSTEREC-
TOMY)
PARA-. . . . . by, beside,
or

modified...(PARANOIA)
(PARAPLEGIA)
(PARATHYROID)
PER -(L)........ .through... (PERFORATE)
(PERMEATE)
PERI-............around....(PERICARDIUM)
(PERISTALSIS)
PLURI-...........many.....(PLURIGLANDULAR)
(PLURILOCULAR)
POLY-...........many or
excessive.. (POLYARTHRITIS)
(POLYGRAPH)
POST-(L).........after......(POSTPARTUM)
(POST-OPERATIVE)
PRE-, PRO-(L).....before.... (PRENATAL)
(PROTHROMBIN)
PSEUDO-..........false......(PSEUDOPOD)
(PSEUDOCYST)
RE-.............again.....(RELAPSE)
(REPRODUCE)
(REINFECT)
RE-, RETRO-(L)....back or
behind.... (REDUCTION)
(RETROPERITONEAL)
SEMI-(L).........half......(SEMILUNAR)
(SEMICOMA)
SINISTR(O)-.......left.......(SINISTROCARDIAL)
SUB-(L)..........under.....(SUBCUTANEOUS)
(SUBCOSTAL)
SUPER-(L)........above or
excessively.(SUPERNUMERARY)
(SUPERIOR)
SUPRA-(L)........above or
upon..... (SUPRACLAVICULAR)
(SUPRAORBITAL)

SYM-, SYN-. . . . . .with or
                          together. . . (SYMPHYSIS)
                                       (SYNCOPE)
                                       (SYNDROME)
TEL-. . . . . end or afar.(TELANGIECTASIA)
                                       (TELEPATHY)
TRANS-(L) . . . . across. . . . .(TRANSFUSION)
                                     (TRANSPOSITION)
UNI-, MON(O)-(L) . . one. . . . . . .(UNILATERAL)
                                     (MONOCYTE)

COMMON SUFFIXES AND
COMBINING TERMS

-AC, -AL, -AN . . . . pertaining
　　　　　　　　　　　to . . . .(ILIAC)
　　　　　　　　　　　　　　　　　(DIGITAL)
　　　　　　　　　　　　　　　　　(OVARIAN)
-AGOGUE . . . . to bear off,
　　　　　　　　　　　carry away .(CHOLAGOGUE)
　　　　　　　　　　　　　　　　　(EMMENAGOGUE)
-ALG(IA),
　-ALGES(IS) . . . . . . pain . . . . . .(NEURALGIA)
　　　　　　　　　　　　　　　　　(ANALGESIC)
-ASE . . . . indicates
　　　　　　　　　　　an enzyme. (AMYLASE)
　　　　　　　　　　　　　　　　　(LIPASE)
　　　　　　　　　　　　　　　　　(PROTEASE)
-ASIS, -OSIS . . . . condition
　　　　　　　　　　　of being. . .(AMEBIASIS)
　　　　　　　　　　　　　　　　　(NEPHROSIS)
-BLAST . . . . germ,
　　　　　　　　　　　sprout or
　　　　　　　　　　　parent of
　　　　　　　　　　　mature cell .(LYMPHOBLAST)
　　　　　　　　　　　　　　　　　(FIBROBLAST)
-CELE . . . . tumor,
　　　　　　　　　　　hernia or
　　　　　　　　　　　swelling. . .(CYSTOCELE)
　　　　　　　　　　　　　　　　　(HYDROCELE)
-CENTESIS . . . . .puncture. . .(PARACENTESIS)

29

		(THORACENTESIS)
-DESIS	a binding	(ARTHRODESIS)
-ECTASIS, -ECTASIA	dilatation or enlargement	(GASTRECTASIS)
		(PHLEBECTASIA)
-ECTOMY	excision of	(APPENDECTOMY)
		(ORCHIDECTOMY)
-FUGE	put to flight	(CENTRIFUGE)
		(FEBRIFUGE)
-GRAPH(Y), -GRAM	writing, describing or record	(CHOLECYSTO-GRAPHY)
		(ELECTROCARDIO-GRAM)
-IA, -Y, -ITY	expression of quality or being	(HYPERCALCEMIA)
		(ATONY)
		(ACIDITY)
-ICLE, -ICULE	expressing diminutive	(PEDICLE)
		(VESICULE)
-ICIAN, -IST, -OR	one who practices	(PHYSICIAN)
		(PHYSIOTHERAPIST)
		(CHIROPRACTOR)
-ITIS	inflammation of	(ENCEPHALITIS)
		(SINUSITIS)
-MALACIA	softening	(OSTEOMALACIA)
		(ENCEPHALO-MALACIA)

-MANIA . . . . madness . . . (MANIAC)
                                  (KLEPTOMANIA)

-ODYN(IA)(E) . . . . . pain . . . . . . (COCCYGODYNIA)
                                  (ANODYNE)

-OID; [-IFORM-L] . . . . like . . . . . . (CARCINOID)
                                  (ENSIFORM)

-(O)LOGY . . . . discourse,
                     science or
                     study of . . . (BACTERIOLOGY)
                                  (PROCTOLOGY)

-OL(E)(US),
  -UL(E)(US) . . . . . expressing
                     diminutive . (ARTERIOLE)
                                  (BRONCHIOLUS)
                                  (VENULE)

-OMA . . . . growth or
                     tumor of . . (SARCOMA)
                                  (NEUROMA)

-OSE . . . . indicates
                     a carbo-
                     hydrate . . . (DEXTROSE)
                                  (LACTOSE)

-OSTOMY . . . . making a
                     mouth or
                     opening
                     into . . . . . . (ENTEROSTOMY)
                                  (COLOSTOMY)

-PEN(IA) . . . . poverty of . (LEUCOPENIA)
                                  (NEUTROPENIA)

-PEXY . . . . fixation
                     of, or
                     fastening . . (OMENTOPEXY)
                                  (NEPHROPEXY)

-PHIL(E)(IA) . . . . . . love, fond-
                     ness for or

```
                          tendency to (HETEROPHILE)
                                      (NEUTROPHILIA)
-PHOB(E)(IA)...... fear of.... (HELIOPHOBE)
                               (HYDROPHOBIA)
-PLASTY........... repair..... (HERNIOPLASTY)
                               (RHINOPLASTY)
-PTOSIS........... falling or
                   dropping of (VISCEROPTOSIS)
                               (NEPHROPTOSIS)
-(R)RHAG(E)(IA).. flowing of. (HEMORRHAGE)
                              (MENORRHAGIA)
-(R)RHAPHY....... sewing of.. (HERNIORRHAPHY)
                              (PHLEBORRHAPHY)
-(R)RHEA......... discharge.. (GONORRHEA)
                              (DYSMENORRHEA)
-(O)SCOP(E)(Y)... inspection,
                  or looking
                  into...... (ESOPHAGOSCOPE)
                             (ENDOSCOPY)
-(O)TOM(E)(Y)....cutting
                  (into).... (MICROTOME)
                             (NEPHROTOMY)
```

COMBINING TERMS -GRAPH (Y), -GRAM, -(O) SCOPE AND -(O) SCOPY

T HE COMBINING terms -GRAPY(Y) and -GRAM (meaning *writing, describing* or *record*) alter the meaning of the same root in medical terms as they do in English words. For example, the TELEGRAPH is the instrument and TELEGRAPHY, the process used in sending messages by wire; while the TELEGRAM is the actual record (or writing) of the message.

Similarly, the ELECTROCARDIOGRAPH is the instrument and ELECTROCARDIOGRAPHY, the process used in recording the electrical impulses (small voltages) due to the beating heart; while the ELECTROCARDIO-GRAM is the actual record (or writing) obtained.

The same principle applies to many such pairs of medical terms indicating either the instrument or the process and the record thereof, such as:

CHOLECYSTOGRAPHY . . . . CHOLECYSTOGRAM
ENCEPHALOGRAPH(Y) . . . . .ENCEPHALOGRAM
UROGRAPHY . . . . UROGRAM
ROENTGENOGRAPHY . . . . .ROENTGENOGRAM
BRONCHOGRAPHY . . . . .BRONCHOGRAM
VENOGRAPHY . . . . VENOGRAM
SPLENOGRAPHY . . . . SPLENOGRAM
CHOLANGIOGRAPHY . . . . CHOLANGIOGRAM
ARTERIOGRAPH(Y) . . . . .ARTERIOGRAM
PLETHSYMOGRAPH(Y) . . . . .PLETHYSMOGRAM
KYMOGRAPH(Y) . . . . .KYMOGRAM
SPHYGMOGRAPH(Y) . . . . .SPHYGMOGRAM

33

The combining term -(O)SCOPY, meaning *looking into* or *inspection,* is found in many words. ENDO-SCOPY, literally meaning *looking into,* is the general term describing all the procedures in which an instrument (term ending in -SCOPE) is used to look into some cavity or tubular structure of the body. For example, the ANOSCOPE is the instrument used to look into the ANUS in the procedure known as ANOSCOPY. Other common procedures and the organs looked into (inspected) are:

BRONCHOSCOPY..........the bronchi
(plural of bronchus)
ESOPHAGOSCOPY.........the esophagus
CYSTOSCOPY............the urinary bladder
GASTROSCOPY...........the stomach
LARYNGOSCOPY..........the larynx
OPHTHALMOSCOPY.......the interior of the eye
OTOSCOPY..............the external ear
PERITONEOSCOPY........the peritoneal cavity
PROCTOSCOPY...........the rectum
SIGMOIDOSCOPY.........the sigmoid colon

A SPECULUM (from the Latin, meaning *mirror*) is the name of an instrument also used to examine the interior of a body cavity (after it dilates its opening). There is a special speculum for ANAL, AURAL, NASAL and VAGINAL examinations, respectively.

PLURAL FORMS OF LATIN NOUNS

W<small>HEN THE</small> singular ends in U<small>M</small>, e.g., S<small>EPTUM</small>, O<small>VUM</small>, D<small>IVERTICULUM</small>; the plural ends in A; (S<small>EPTA</small>, O<small>VA</small>, D<small>IVERTICULA</small>).

When the singular ends in U<small>S</small>, e.g., F<small>UNDUS</small>, U<small>TERUS</small>, C<small>OCCUS</small>; the plural ends in I; (F<small>UNDI</small>, U<small>TERI</small>, C<small>OCCI</small>). Exception is V<small>ISCUS</small>, the plural being V<small>ISCERA</small>.

When the singular ends in I<small>X</small>, e.g., A<small>PPENDIX</small>, V<small>ARIX</small>, C<small>ERVIX</small>; the plural ends in I<small>CES</small>; (A<small>PPENDICES</small>, V<small>ARICES</small>, C<small>ERVICES</small>).

When the singular ends in I<small>S</small>, e.g., C<small>IRRHOSIS</small>, T<small>ESTIS</small>; the plural ends in E<small>S</small>; (C<small>IRRHOSES</small>, T<small>ESTES</small>).

Certain words ending in I<small>TIS</small>, e.g., A<small>RTHRITIS</small>, M<small>YO-CARDITIS</small>, E<small>NDOCARDITIS</small>; end in I<small>DITES</small> in their plural forms; (A<small>RTHRIDITES</small>, M<small>YOCARDIDITES</small>, E<small>NDOCARDI-DITES</small>).

When the singular ends in A, e.g., U<small>VULA</small>, U<small>RETHRA</small>, F<small>ASCIA</small>; the plural ends in A<small>E</small>; (U<small>VULAE</small>, U<small>RETHRAE</small>, F<small>ASCIAE</small>).

Certain nouns derived from the Greek, such as S<small>TIGMA</small>, S<small>TOMA</small>, C<small>ARCINOMA</small> and T<small>RAUMA</small> end in A<small>TA</small> in their plural forms (S<small>TIGMATA</small>, S<small>TOMATA</small>, C<small>ARCI-NOMATA</small> and T<small>RAUMATA</small>) although the modern forms S<small>TIGMAS</small>, S<small>TOMAS</small>, C<small>ARCINOMAS</small> and T<small>RAUMAS</small> are also acceptable and perhaps preferable.

SOME MEDICAL TERMS OF PURE LATIN

PER OS, literally *by way of* or *through the mouth*, refers to method of administering medication.

COR BOVINUM, literally *ox heart*, is the term used to describe the markedly hypertrophied (enlarged) heart seen in advanced aortic valvular disease of the heart.

ANGINA PECTORIS, literally severe *oppression or constriction of the chest*, is the well known symptom of coronary insufficiency with MYOCARDIAL ISCHEMIA (from the Greek ISCH, *to check or cut down* and -EMIA, *blood*).

IN SITU, literally means *in position* or *place*. Its derived meanings are *in a given or natural position* or *undisturbed*.

STATUS ANGINOSIS, STATUS ASTHMATICUS and STATUS EPILEPTICUS are used to describe the continuous state of constricting chest pains, asthma and epilepsy, respectively.

THROMBOANGIITIS OBLITERANS (also called BUERGER'S DISEASE) is an inflammatory and obliterative disease of the blood vessels of the extremities, usually the lower, occurring chiefly in young and middle-aged males.

SITUS INVERSUS, literally *altered position,* is the term used to describe the rare ANOMALY (from the Greek ANOMALIA, meaning *deviation from the usual*) in which the organs are changed from the normal to the opposite side of the body. The condition is also known as TRANSPOSITION of the VISCERA.

GENU VALGUM ("KNOCK-KNEE") and GENU VARUM ("BOW-LEG") refer to the deformities of the knee (GENU,) in which it is turned inward (VALGUM) or outward (VARUM), respectively.

ARCUS SENILIS, literally *arch of senility,* is the arched opacity surrounding the cornea of the eye, seen in the aged.

HALLUX VALGUS ("BUNION") and HALLUX VARUS refer to the deformities of the big toe (HALLUX), which is deviated inward or outward, respectively.

COXA VALGA and COXA VARA refer to deformities of the hip joint (COXA) with increase or decrease of the angulation of the neck of the femur with its shaft, respectively.

PES PLANUS, literally and actually means *flatfoot.*

DELIRIUM TREMENS refers to a delirious state accompanied by constant tremors and severe exhaustion, associated with alcoholic intoxication.

DIABETES MELLITUS, usually referred to as just DIABETES, is a metabolic disturbance characterized by excessive thirst, excessive amount of urinary output and the presence of sugar in the urine and blood. DIABETES INSIPIDUS is due to a disorder of the hypothalamus and is similar to diabetes mellitus except for the absence of sugar in the urine and blood.

The terms FETUS, PELVIS, RECTUM, PATELLA, ANGINA and VAGINA are examples of pure Latin words adopted into English.

LOCUM TENENS, literally *holding the place,* is used to describe a substitute or temporary practitioner carrying on a practice during the absence of the regular physician.

LOCOMOTOR ATAXIA, literally *unsteadiness of locomotion,* is the old term for TABES DORSALIS, a degenerative neurological disease dependent upon sclerosis of the dorsal (posterior) columns of the spinal cord, due to syphilis.

MATERIA MEDICA, literally meaning *medical matter,* refers to the list of agents used for therapeutic purposes. The term is also used to denote that branch of medicine dealing with drugs, their composition, dosages, methods of use, etc.

SOME MEDICAL TERMS DERIVED FROM MYTHOLOGY

APHRODISIAC, from APHRODITE, the Greek goddess of love.

EROTIC, from EROS, a Greek god of love.

HERMAPHRODITE, the name of the son of Hermes and Aphrodite, is the medical term indicating an individual having both male and female genitals.

HYGIENE, from HYGEIA, the goddess of health, one of the daughters of Aesculapius, the god of medicine.

MORPHINE, from MORPHEUS, the god of dreams.

PANACEA, meaning a *cure-all*, is the name of another daughter of Aesculapius.

VENEREAL, from VENUS, Roman goddess of love. [VENUS, VENERIS-L]

NARCISSISM, meaning *self-love*, from NARCISSUS, who was in love with his own image reflected in water. Narcissus, a spring flower that grows near water, is also named after the same mythological character.

OEDIPUS COMPLEX is used in psychiatry to describe a young man's perverted love of his mother accompanied by a hatred for his father, based on a mythological story.

CAPUT MEDUSAE literally means *the head of Medusa*. The latter is a mythological character whose golden hair was turned into snakes by Minerva. The dilated periumbilical collateral veins seen in portal obstruction were so named because of their snake-like appearance.

PRIAPISM, from PRIAPUS, the god of procreation.

PSYCHE, meaning *spirit* or *mind*, from PSYCHE, the lover of Cupid.

SATYRIASIS, meaning *male beastliness*, from SATYR, a woodland demon, half animal and half man and follower of Bacchus, the god of wine.

ATLAS, the first (uppermost) cervical vertebra supporting the skull, was named after ATLAS, the mythological giant (a Titan), who supported the heavens on his shoulders.

PROTEAN, meaning *taking on many forms or shapes*, from PROTEUS, a sea god, who assumed different shapes when seized.

ATROPINE, an alkaloid obtained from the plant ATROPA BELLADONNA was named after ATROPOS, one of the three Fates, who "cut the thread of life." The latter activity explains the selection of the name for this poisonous plant.

TENDO ACHILLIS or ACHILLES TENDON, the tendon of the heel (CALCANEUS), was named after ACHILLES, a Greek legendary hero. He was dipped into the river Styx by his mother, Thetis, thus making him invulnerable. As the heel, by which she held him, was not submerged, it was vulnerable to a mortal wound inflicted upon it by Paris.

IRIS, the circular colored membrane surrounding the pupil of the eye, was named after IRIS, goddess of the rainbow and messenger of the gods. The term, meaning *a rainbow* in Greek, is also applied to a group of plants with vari-colored flowers.

HEBE, the goddess of youth, is the origin of the term HEBEPHRENIA, meaning *adolescent insanity*, a form of dementia precox.

HELIOS, the Greek sun-god and meaning *sun*, is the origin of many terms as: HELIUM, the gaseous element, so named because it was discovered in the sun's atmosphere; HELIOTHERAPY, treatment by sun baths; HELIOTROPE, any plant which turns toward the sun; HELIOPHOBIA, morbid fear of exposure to the sun's rays, etc.

SOME MEDICAL TERMS DERIVED FROM HISTORY

CESAREAN (or CAESARIAN) SECTION was so named because Julius Caesar is alleged to have been delivered in this manner.

LESBIANISM is derived from LESBOS, a greek island in the Aegean, the home of Sappho, who was addicted to this perversion.

SADISM was named after the Marquis de Sade (1740-1814), who practiced this perversion.

MASOCHISM derives its name from the Austrian novelist SACHER-MASOCH (1836-1895), who first described this perversion, which is the reverse of sadism.

NICOTINE, the alkaloid in tobacco, was so named after JEAN NICOT, who first brought tobacco to France in 1560.

SYPHILIS, the name of a venereal disease, is believed to be derived from a famous medical poem by Fracastro published in Venice in 1530, titled "Syphilis sive Morbus Gallicus." SYPHILIS (meaning a *swineherd*) was the name of one of the poem's characters who acquired the disease. The poem recognized the venereal cause of syphilis and reviewed the then current knowledge concerning it. The title of the poem implied that the disease was French in origin. A common custom in those days was for each country to blame the other for introducing the disease; the French called it the Neapolitan disease; the Russians called it the Polish disease; the Persians called it the Turkish disease, and so on. Even Columbus' sailors were blamed for bringing the disease to Europe from America. LUES (originally expressed as LUES VENERA), meaning *pestilence* in Latin, is an alternative term for syphilis. The disease was also known as the POX, the GREAT POX, the FRENCH POX and the SPANISH POX.

MESMERISM (and its verb MESMERIZE), named after FRIEDRICH ANTON MESMER (1734-1815), a German physician, began as a cross between the concepts of astrology and those of the then recently discovered electricity and magnetism. At first Mesmer stroked his patients with magnets, later with his hands, in the false belief that he was effecting a "cure" by endowing them with some mysterious force he called "animal magnetism."

FLETCHERISM was named after HORACE FLETCHER (1849-1919), an American dietitian who was fanatic in his insistence that food should be taken in definite quantities, at definite times, most thoroughly and minutely masticated and swallowed with sips of water, His theory, an obviously absurd exaggeration of certain sound hygienic dietary principles, was soon relegated to oblivion.

SOME MEDICAL TERMS CONTAINING PROPER NAMES (EPONYMS)

MANY MEDICAL TERMS contain the proper names of persons who first described or discovered an anatomical part, a symptom, sign, test, syndrome, or condition. These terms are known as EPONYMS, examples of which are HORNER'S SYNDROME, ROMBERG'S SIGN, HIRSCHSPRUNG'S DISEASE, EUSTACHIAN TUBE, WASSERMANN TEST, POUPART'S LIGAMENT, GRAVE'S DISEASE, BARANY'S SIGN, SIMS' POSITION, RORSCHACH TEST, and many others too numerous to list here. However, the modern scientific trend is to discontinue the use of proper names in medical nomenclature in spite of the fact that many of these are firmly entrenched, especially in the minds of older physicians and scientists.

Exceptions are certain universally accepted terms incorporating proper names, such as ROENTGENOLOGY, PASTEURIZATION, CURIE, AMPERE, FREUDIAN, GALVANOMETER, SADISM, BRUCELLOSIS, etc., as well as certain established eponyms, such as MECKEL'S DIVERTICULUM, AMPULLA OF VATER, HODGKIN'S DISEASE, FROHLICH'S SYNDROME, SCHICK TEST, DICK TEST, BANTI'S DISEASE, etc., for which non-eponym terms are either too complicated, confusing or perhaps as yet unavailable.

Many bacteria are named after physicians or other scientists. The stories behind the names make interesting reading. Only a few highlights will be mentioned here.

RICKETTSIA, a class of organisms found in TYPHUS FEVER, TRENCH FEVER and ROCKY MOUNTAIN SPOTTED FEVER, was named after HOWARD TAYLOR RICKETTS (1871-1910), an American pathologist.

BRUCELLA, the bacillus that causes BRUCELLOSIS (UNDULANT or MALTA FEVER), was named after DAVID BRUCE (1855-1931), British pathologist and bacteriologist.

PASTEURELLA, a genus of bacteria, was named after the famous French scientist and bacteriologist, LOUIS PASTEUR (1822-1895). PASTEURELLA PESTIS (the plague bacillus) and PASTEURELLA TULARENSIS (the causative agent of TULAREMIA) are two of its many species. Incidentally, TULAREMIA (rabbit fever), a disease of rodents, transmitted by the bites of insects and acquired by man through handling of the infected animals, was named after TULARE COUNTY, CALIFORNIA, where it was first described.

SALMONELLA, a group of bacteria, one of the causes of acute gastroenteritis of food poisoning, was named after DANIEL ELMER SALMON (1850-1914), an American pathologist. Many types of SALMONELLA are designated by names of cities, hospitals, and patients related to their discovery.

NEISSERIA, a genus of anaerobic GRAM negative cocci, was named after ALBERT NEISSER (1855-1916), a German physician who, in 1879, discovered the GONOCOCCUS, the cause of gonorrhea. In 1906, in collaboration with WASSERMANN and BRUCK, he introduced the specific blood test (WASSERMANN TEST) in the detection of syphilis. The literal meaning of the term GONORRHEA is a *discharge of semen,* thus reflecting the erroneous concept of this disease by the ancients, who mistook the pus for semen.

LISTERIA or LISTERELLA a genus of bacteria, was named after JOSEPH LISTER (1827-1912), an English surgeon, who introduced the use of antiseptics in the operating room and thus is known as the founder of antiseptic surgery. He also has a proprietary antiseptic solution named after him.

FINLAYA, a subgenus of AEDES mosquitoes which transmit yellow fever, was named after CARLOS FINLAY (1833-1915), a Cuban biologist and physician, who, in 1881, postulated the theory that yellow fever is transmitted to man by mosquitoes. Some years later (1901) Walter Reed (1851-1902), an American Army surgeon, published evidence that yellow fever is caused by a filterable virus transmitted to man by a mosquito (AEDES AEGYPTI), thus proving Finlay's theory.

GRAM'S STAIN, an important, commonly used stain, differentiating bacteria into Gram positive and Gram negative groups, is named after its originator, HANS CHRISTIAN GRAM (1853-1938), a Danish bacteriologist.

ONOMATOPOETIC WORDS

THE TERM ONOMATOPOETIC is derived from the Greek ONOMA, meaning *a name* and POIEIN, meaning *made*, and thus means *a made name*. Onomatopoetic words, when spoken, are intended to reproduce specific sounds and are therefore sometimes described as "echoic" words. Examples are *belch, hiccup, retch, borborygmus,* (audible sounds caused by rumbling intestinal gases), *murmur, tympany, rale, croup, gargle,* and certain, once respectable, four letter words.

The term QUACK, when referred to a "healer," (usually not a member of the legitimate professions), is probably an echoic word imitating the sound of the loud quacking of a duck. It is believed to connote the boastfulness of the unethical or illegal practitioner in praising himself, his methods of treatment or his remedies.

INTERESTING DERIVATIONS OF SOME MEDICAL WORDS

LUMEN (L), meaning *light;* hence something which transmits light, that is, a clear space such as the interior of hollow organs or tubular structures as blood vessels, ducts, etc.

JEJUNUM (L), meaning *empty,* was the name given to the upper small intestine because the ancient anatomists found it empty after death.

CECUM (L), meaning *blind,* refers to the first portion of the large intestine so named because it has a blind end.

FOCUS (L), meaning *fireplace,* hence its modern meaning, *the center of light and heat.*

HYSTERIA, from the Greek HYSTERA, meaning *womb,* is defined as the manifestation of symptoms of purely functional origin, based on the ancient erroneous belief that the cause of functional or nervous disorders was disease of the uterus.

HYPOCHONDRIA, derived from the Greek, literally means a *condition below the cartilages,* that is, in the pit of the stomach or epigastrium. Because of the frequency of alleged pains in this region complained of by patients with nervous disorders, the term is used to describe this functional (non-organic) condition.

VACCINATION is derived from the Latin word VACCA, meaning *cow.*

BERI-BERI is an Asiatic word meaning *extreme weak-*

ness, the chief symptom in the vitamin (thiamine) deficiency disease so named.

IDIOT, derived from the Greek, literally means *a private person or citizen* (as distinguished from one holding public office). The meaning of the term gradually changed until it came to mean *an individual with the lowest grade of mental deficiency, usually congenital.*

THORAX, derived from the Greek, meaning *breast plate,* now refers to the chest, which is covered by the breast plate.

NAUSEA, derived from the Greek word NAUS, meaning *ship,* whence its modern meaning *sick to the stomach,* based on the original reference to sea-sickness. The English word NAUTICAL has the same derivation.

PYLORUS, derived from the Greek word PYLOROS, meaning *gatekeeper,* and is thus the medical term applied to the *stomach outlet.*

PHYSICS, PHYSICIAN, PHYSICIST and PHYSICAL are all derived from the Greek word PHYSIS, meaning *nature.*

ORTHOPEDICS is derived from the Greek ORTHOS, *straight,* and PED, *child,* and originally referred to that branch of medical practice concerned with the correction of deformities in children. The term later came to include adults.

HYDROPHOBIA, the older term for RABIES, *madness,* literally means *fear of water,* so named because the ancient Greeks noted that the sufferer was afraid to drink because it caused a violent spasm of the throat muscles.

PARASITE, derived from the Greek, literally means *taking food by the side of.* Later it came to mean *eating at the table of another.* Its derived meaning is *living off another,* as applied to organisms.

SYMPOSIUM in ancient Greece meant a *drinking party with some intellectual conversation.* Now it means a *conference with intellectual conversation — but no drinking.*

ECLAMPSIA, the name of a serious form of toxemia of pregnancy, is derived from the Greek EKLAMPSIS, meaning *a flash of light,* so named because the sufferers were supposed to see flashes of light during the attacks.

MEDICINE and SCIENCE are derived from the Latin words MEDICINA, meaning *art of healing,* and SCIENTIA, meaning *knowledge,* respectively.

IATROS is a Greek word meaning *physician* or *healing.* Examples of words containing this root are PEDIATRICS, IATROGENIC and IATROCHEMISTRY.

CANCER in Latin means *crab.* CARCINOMA is derived from the Greek CARCIN, also meaning *crab,* and -OMA, meaning *tumor.* Thus the ancients apparently likened malignant tumors to crabs probably because of the similarity of their appearance and spreading tendencies. CANKER originally had the same meaning as cancer, but has come to mean a *benign sore in the mouth.* The term CHANCRE, the *primary sore of syphilis,* also arose from a modification of cancer.

ICTERUS is derived from the Greek word IKTEROS, meaning *a yellow bird.* It is synonymous with JAUNDICE (from the French JAUNISSE, meaning *yellowness*) and either term is used to describe the yellowish discoloration of the skin and mucous membranes due to bile pigments in the blood.

DUODENUM in Latin means *twelve.* This, the first portion of the small intestine, was so named by the ancients because they estimated it to be twelve fingerbreadth's in length.

CHOLERA literally means *a flow of bile*. Because of the profuse outpouring of bile and bile-like fluids, both orally and rectally, the ancient Greeks so named this acute, infectious, specific, epidemic disease characterized by severe diarrhea, vomiting and collapse.

CHOLESTERIN, literally *solid bile*, was so named because gall stones (of the cholesterin variety) were thought to be solidified bile. Actually, CHOL-ESTERIN (or CHOLESTEROL, the more correct term) is a complex alcohol of the class of *sterols*, highly important in metabolism and found, not only in certain gall stones, but in animal fats and oils, bile, blood, nerve tissue and egg yolk.

LUNACY, from the Latin word LUNA, meaning *moon*, literally means *moon-sickness*. Its modern equivalent is INSANITY.

THERAPY and THERAPEUTICS are derived from the Greek word THERAPEUEIN, meaning *to heal* or *to take care of*. Examples of the many combined forms are PHYSIOTHERAPY, CHEMOTHERAPY, RADIOTHERAPY, PHARMACOTHERAPY, PSYCHO-THERAPY, BALNEOTHERAPY, HELIOTHERAPY, DIETOTHERAPY, etc.

SURGERY is the shortened form of the Old English term CHIRURGERY, which is derived from the Greek words CHIR, meaning *hand*, and ERGON, meaning *work;* thus, *to work by hand*. Some British universities still award a special surgical degree, B.Ch., or B.Chir. (Bachelor of Surgery).

ARTERY is derived from the Greek word ARTERIA which

is the combination of AER, meaning *air*, and TERRO, meaning *carry;* so named by the ancients in their erroneous belief that the arteries contained air during life because they were found empty after death.

BELLADONNA means *beautiful lady* in Italian. The drug was so named because of the popular belief that the ladies of Italy used it to make their eyes more beautiful by its action of dilating the pupils.

MELANCHOLIA literally means a *condition of black bile*, erroneously believed by the ancients to be the cause of *mental depression*, the modern derived meaning of the term.

MALARIA, literally meaning *bad air*, was so named because the disease was thought to be caused thereby.

HEMOPHILIA, from the Greek, meaning *tendency to bleed*, is a hereditary blood disease occurring in males (transmitted by females) characterized by delayed clotting of the blood and thus an uncontrollable tendency to hemorrhage. The condition is mentioned in the TALMUD as an acceptable excuse for omitting circumcision in instances of a family history of this disease.

PODAGRA, from the Greek meaning *a seizure of the foot*, is another name for GOUT, so named by the ancients who recognized the characteristic symptom of the disease, namely, a sudden attack of severe pain in the big toe.

CADUCEUS, meaning *herald's staff* in Latin, refers to the staff carried by Mercury, the messenger of the gods (in Greek mythology). This staff, with *two serpents* twined about it, their heads meeting at the top, and bearing wings, became the symbol of public office carried by Roman heralds. In modern times it has become the insignia of the Medical Corps of the United States Army, being its administrative emblem implying neutrality and non-combattant status. The authentic insignia of MEDICINE, however, consists of the staff of Aesculapius about which a *single serpent* is coiled, thus distinguishing it from the original non-medical caduceus of Mercury with which it is often confused.

OBESITY is derived from the Latin OBESUS, meaning *eaten up or lean.* This original meaning gradually was changed to its present (and opposite)) meaning, namely *overweight.* A better term, perhaps, would be ADIPOSITY or ADIPOSIS (from the Latin ADEPS, ADIP(IS), *fat*).

NURSE is derived from the Latin NUTRIX, *a nurse* (from NUTRIRE, *to suckle or nourish*). The term became NOURICE (French), then NURICE (middle English) and finally NURSE in modern English. The original meaning of "one who suckles, nourishes or cares for an infant" has become "one who cares for any sick or helpless person."

SIAMESE TWINS originally referred to an instance of double monstrosity in the persons of famous twins (1814-1874) born in Siam (of Chinese extraction), who were united between the xiphoid cartilages by a thick fleshy ligament. The term is now used to describe any double monster (conjoined twins).

LONGEVITY, from the Latin LONGAEVITAS, meaning *long life,* has come to usually mean "length of life." Thanks to the phenomenal advances in modern medical sciences, both preventive and therapeutic, the term is assuming its original meaning. For example, a baby born in 1956 has a life expectancy of 73 years as compared to only 51 years for a baby born in 1900. The many thousands of healthy and happy people over 60 years of age will be amused at this, the ancient Romans' conception of the AGES of MAN:

PUERITIA..........Childhood (to 5 years)
ADOLESCENTIA......Youth (to 18 years)
JUVENTUS.........Young man (to 25 years)
MAJORES..........Man (25 to 50 years)
SENECTUS.........Old man (50 to 60 years)
CREPITA AETAS.....Decrepit old age (60 years to death)

DOCTOR, from the Latin DOCTUS, meaning *teacher,* is a title applied to many persons, both in and out of the healing professions. Its original connotation is still retained in the many academic degrees (DOCTORATES) signifying competence in a special branch of learning. It is also used in honorary degrees awarded by universities to individuals who have distinguished themselves in various fields of human endeavor.

Following is a list of academic degrees containing the title DOCTOR: (The source of information for those outside the healing professions is the American Council on Education.)

*D.C............Doctor of Chiropractic
D.C.E..........Doctor of Civil Engineering
D.C.L..........Doctor of Civil Law
D.C.S..........Doctor of Commercial Science
D.D............Doctor of Divinity
*D.D.S..........Doctor of Dental Surgery
D.Ed...........Doctor of Education

*D.M.D......... Doctor of Dental Medicine
D.M.L......... Doctor of Modern Languages
D.M.S. or
   Med. Sc. D.... Doctor of Medical Science
*D.O........... Doctor of Osteopathy
D.P.H......... Doctor of Public Health
D.R.E......... Doctor of Religious Education
D. Sc......... Doctor of Science
*D.S.C........ Doctor of Surgical Chiropody
*D.V.M........ Doctor of Veterinary Medicine
HH. D......... Doctor of Humanities
L.H.D......... Doctor of Humane Letters
LL. D......... Doctor of Laws
*M.D.......... Doctor of Medicine
*O.D.......... Doctor of Optometry
Phar. D....... Doctor of Pharmacy
Ph. D......... Doctor of Philosophy
S.Sc.D........ Doctor of Social Sciences
S.T.D......... Doctor of Sacred Theology

*Degrees applied to members of the healing professions.

The literal and original meanings of some terms differ from their actual and modern meanings. AS-PHYXIA, literally *no pulse*, has come to mean *suffocation*. LITHOTOMY, literally *cutting into stone*, really should be LITHECTOMY, as the operation consists of the removal of the stone from the body. The same applies to VAGOTOMY in which operation portions of the vagus nerve are excised. The term should therefore be replaced by VAGECTOMY, which correction is noted more and more in the recent literature. Similarly, OVARIOTOMY should be OVARIECTOMY. NYSTAGMUS, from the Greek, meaning *nodding of the head or drowsiness*, has come to mean *oscillatory movements of the eyeballs*. Fortunately, these misleading terms are few. Long usage and general acceptance have sanctioned their retention in the medical vocabulary. It would be difficult to change or delete them in spite of their recognized confusing and unscientific attributes.

ROOTS AND WORDS OFTEN CONFUSED BECAUSE OF SIMILARITY IN SOUND OR SPELLING

ORAL, referring to the *mouth*; and AURAL, referring to the *ear*.

MY(O), meaning *muscle*; and MYEL(O); meaning *marrow*.

-CELE, the combining term meaning a *tumor, hernia,* or *swelling*; and CELI(O) or COELI(O), meaning *belly, abdomen,* or *any cavity* or *hollow of the body*.

BLAST, meaning *cell* or *sprout*; and PLAST, meaning *mold*.

ILEUM, meaning *lower small intestine*; and ILIUM(L), meaning *hip bone*.

MENS-(L), meaning *mind*; and MENS(ES), meaning *menstrual flow*.

OS, ORIS-(L), meaning *mouth*; and OS, OSSIS-(L), meaning *bone*.

PALPATION-(L), meaning *manual examination;* and PALPITATION-(L), meaning consciousness of one's *heart action*.

PES, PEDIS-(L), meaning *foot;* and PED, meaning *child*.

EPIDEMIC, ENDEMIC and PANDEMIC are all derived from the Greek word DEM(OS), meaning *people*. A disease is EPIDEMIC when it occurs in outbreaks; ENDEMIC when it is always present in a country or region; PANDEMIC when it occurs simultaneously in many countries.

PROTEIN, the *important food constituent;* and PROTEAN, meaning *taking on many forms or shapes.*

UTERUS, the *womb*; and URETERS, the *long narrow tubes conveying urine from the kidneys to the urinary bladder,* may be confused with each other if hastily spoken or carelessly written.

MENORRHAGIA, literally *monthly flowing,* meaning an *excessive monthly (menstrual) flow;* and METRORRHAGIA, literally *uterine flowing,* meaning *uterine hemorrhage independent of the menstrual period.*

PERITONEUM, the *lining of the abdominal cavity and the covering of its viscera;* and PERINEUM, *the region anterior to the anus.*

CERVICAL, the adjective form of the noun CERVIX, meaning *neck,* usually refers to the neck of the uterus (CERVIX UTERI); it may also refer to the neck portion of the spine (CERVICAL VERTEBRAE).

SOME INCORRECTLY USED EXPRESSIONS

LISTED ARE SOME common expressions incorrectly used mostly by the layman, but occasionally by the careless professional person. The student and worker in the medical and allied fields should be familiar with them so as to avoid them himself and tactfully correct them when perpetrated by others.

It will suffice to merely mention here the numerous, and often humorous, errors due to plain ignorance of the English language, such as: *ulster* for *ulcer, bronical* for *bronchial, bulge* for *belch, prostrate* for *prostate, enemy* for *enema, chronical* for *chronic, larnyx* for *larynx,* etc.

The characteristic, and sometimes picturesque, jargon of the medical profession is tolerable and harmless as long as it is kept within the confines of the profession. There is no intent to condemn or censor the intimate conversation among professional colleagues. However, the use of incorrect English by anyone, especially the professional person, is in poor taste and inexcusable. Besides, it is jarring to the sensibilities of the listener or reader.

COLITIS, meaning *inflammation of the colon,* implies an organic disease and the term should, therefore, be applied only to the organic diseases, ULCERATIVE COLITIS, AMEBIC COLITIS and BACILLARY DYSENTERY. The conditions commonly known as SPASTIC COLITIS and MUCOUS COLITIS are incorrectly named as they are not organic diseases. Both are functional (nervous) disorders and should properly be called SPASTIC COLON or IRRITABLE COLON. A further reason for deploring the use of the term COLITIS in these functional conditions is that the already apprehensive and nervous patient is made worse by the connotation of this mis-leading term.

TEMPERATURE, *a reading of the number of degrees of heat,* is not synonymous with FEVER. The expression, *"running a temperature"* is therefore meaningless, as everyone alive is doing so. When the temperature is above 100°F. then FEVER (or an ELEVATED TEMPERATURE) is said to be present.

DYSENTERY is a *severe, toxic, bloody diarrhea.* The term, therefore, should not be used to indicate a simple frequency of non-bloody bowel movements, for which the correct term is DIARRHEA.

The expression, "TO OPERATE A CASE" is a glaring example of desecrated English. Obviously it is the PATIENT and not the CASE that is operated on, and not OPERATED.

GASTRITIS, derived from GASTR, *stomach* and ITIS, *inflammation of,* and meaning, *inflammation of (the lining of) the stomach,* does not imply the presence of GAS, in spite of the suggestive sound and spelling of its first syllable.

In modern dentistry a TOOTH is not PULLED but is EXTRACTED.

The stomach is only one of the many organs contained in the ABDOMEN. Many, including some so-called educated people, often erroneously say STOMACH when they mean ABDOMEN, as, for example, in the doleful statement: *"My stomach is getting bigger"!* When a patient states that he has *"pain in the stomach,"* he may

or may not be right. BELLY, synonymous with ABDO-
MEN, is a perfectly respectable word, but for some
unknown reason is looked upon as vulgar.

A formerly common expression, which fortunately
is now only rarely heard, is the vague, unscientific,
though apparently satisfying, diagnosis of *"a touch of
appendicitis, pneumonia, diabetes, or some other disease."* Modern scientific medicine does not tolerate
such ambiguous, irrational, and sometimes artful,
statements.

"YELLOW JAUNDICE", an expression used occasionally by the uninformed, is an obvious redundancy, equivalent to saying "yellow yellowness."

"SUGAR DIABETES" is another example of a redund-
ant expression.

LYMPH GLAND is an obsolete, incorrect term for
LYMPH NODE. A GLAND elaborates and discharges a
secretion or excretion, which a NODE does not do.
LYMPH NODE is therefore the proper term.

When a patient states that he has ULCERS he is most
likely exaggerating in using the plural. More than one
ulcer, though occasionally seen, is very rare. When he
adds that his ulcer is "gastric" or in the "stomach,"
the chances are that he is wrong again, as the common-
est location of PEPTIC ULCER (the generic term for all
ulcers in the digestive tract dependent on the acid-pep-
sin factor) is in the DUODENUM (the first portion of the
small intestine adjacent to the outlet of the stomach).
DUODENAL ULCER is about ten times more common
than GASTRIC ULCER.

The term REGIME is frequently used instead of REGI-
MEN in referring to a system, course or mode of treatment. Although both words are doublets, being derived from the same Latin word REGERE, *to rule,* the

former applies to a system of government or rule. The latter, in correct medical terminology, indicates a set of rules regulating diet, exercise or other therapeutic measures; for example, ULCER REGIMEN.

SOME COMMON LAY EXPRESSIONS DEFINED IN MEDICAL TERMS

"Adam's apple".... The THYROID CARTILAGE of the LARYNX, when prominent.

"afterbirth"........PLACENTA (*a cake*-L)

"air-swallowing"....AEROPHAGIA

"athlete's foot".....DERMATOPHYTOSIS, a form of ringworm infection involving the hands and feet.

"armpit"..........AXILLA-(L)

"artificial teeth";
"plates"........DENTURES

"baldness".......ALOPECIA (from ALOPEX, *fox*)

"barber's itch".....TINEA SYCOSIS, a form of ringworm infection involving the bearded areas.

"barrel chest"......EMPHYSEMATOUS CHEST

"belly button";
"navel".........UMBILICUS-(L)

"bed sore"........DECUBITUS (from DECUMBERE-L, *to lie down*) ULCER

"bed wetting"......ENURESIS (from ENOUREIN, *to make water in*)

"Bell's palsy"......FACIAL NERVE PARALYSIS

"(the) bends".....CRAMPS IN THE EXTREMITIES and ABDOMEN due to CAISSON DISEASE (or COMPRESSED AIR ILLNESS)

"birthmark".......NEVUS (from NAEVUS-L, *mole*)

63

"black and blue". . . ECCHYMOSIS (from EC, *out,*
CHYM(OS), *juice* and OSIS)

"blackhead". . . . . . . COMEDO

"blood poison". . . . . SEPTICEMIA

"boils". . . . . FURUNCULOSIS

"bowleg". . . . . GENU VARUM

"bread pill";
"sugar pill". . . . . . PLACEBO (*I shall please*-L)

"break" (referring
to a bone). . . . . . FRACTURE

"breastbone". . . . . . STERNUM

"bruise". . . . . CONTUSION

"bugs". . . . . BACTERIA (from BAKTERI(ON),
little staff)

"bunion". . . . . HALLUX VALGUS

"(to) burn off". . . . CAUTERIZE (thermally or chemi-
cally)

"burp". . . . . BELCH; ERUCTATION

"chafing". . . . . INTERTRIGO (from INTER, *between* and TRITUM-L, *to rub*)

"change of life". . . . MENOPAUSE; CLIMACTERIC
(from KLIMAKTER, *rung of a
ladder*)

"charleyhorse". . . . . STIFFNESS DUE TO MUSCLE
STRAIN

"chicken pox". . . . . . VARICELLA (from VARI(US)-L,
various)

"clap". . . . . GONORRHEA

"clubfoot". . . . . TALIPES

"cold sore";
"fever blister". . . . HERPES SIMPLEX

"collar bone". . . . . . CLAVICLE

"common cold". . . . ACUTE CORYZA or RHINITIS

"consumption". . . . . TUBERCULOSIS

"corn". . . . . .CLAVUS
"crabs". . . . . .PEDICULOSIS PUBIS
"cross eyes";
   "squint". . . . . STRABISMUS
"croup". . . . . .ACUTE OBSTRUCTIVE LARYNGITIS
"curvature of spine". SCOLIOSIS
"(a) cut". . . . . .A LACERATION
"to cut off". . . . . . . .TO AMPUTATE (usually referring
       to part or all of an extremity, but occasionally
       to part or all of an internal organ.)
"dandruff". . . . . SCALES OF SEBORRHEA CAPITIS
"death of tissue". . . .NECROSIS
"dizziness". . . . . VERTIGO
"dope". . . . . NARCOTICS
"dried up". . . . . .DEHYDRATED
"dropped organs". . .VISCEROPTOSIS
"dropsy". . . . . .EDEMA; ASCITES
"drug rash". . . . . . . DERMATITIS MEDICAMENTOSA
"ear wax". . . . . .CERUMEN (from CERA-L, *wax*)
"excessive appetite". BULIMIA; HYPOREXIA
"fainting";
   "black out". . . . . .SYNCOPE
"falling sickness". . . EPILEPSY
"false pregnancy". . .PSEUDOCYESIS (from PSEUD(ES),
              false and KYESIS, *pregnancy*)
"farsightedness". . . . HYPERMETROPIA
"fever". . . . . PYREXIA
"fingers and toes". . .DIGITS
"fits". . . . . .EPILEPTIC SEIZURES
"flat foot". . . . . .PES PLANUS
"floating kidney". . . NEPHROPTOSIS
"flu; "grippe". . . . . .INFLUENZA
"galloping
   consumption". . . .ACUTE MILIARY TUBERCULOSIS
"gas". . . . . .FLATULENCE

"German measles". . RUBELLA (from RUBELL(US)-L, *reddish*)

"glandular fever". . . INFECTIOUS MONONUCLEOSIS

"goose flesh";

   "goose pimples". . CUTIS ANSERINA (from ANSER-L, *a goose*)

"gravel". . . . . CALCULI (STONES) in gall bladder, kidney or bladder

"graying of hair". . . CANITIES (*hoariness*-L)

"gullet". . . . . ESOPHAGUS

"gum boil". . . . . ALVEOLAR ABSCESS

"habit spasms". . . . . TICS

"hangnail infection";

   "run-a-round". . . . PARONYCHIA (from PARA, *besides* and ONYX, *nail*)

"heartburn". . . . . . . PYROSIS (from PYR(ETUS), *fire* and OSIS)

"high arched foot". . PES CAVUS

"hives". . . . . URTICARIA

"hoarseness". . . . . . . DYSPHONIA

"housemaid's knee". BURSITIS OF KNEE

"humpback" or

   "hunchback". . . . KYPHOSIS

"hydrophobia". . . . . RABIES

"in the family way". PREGNANT

"infantile paralysis";

   "polio". . . . . ANTERIOR POLIOMYELITIS

"irritable heart";

   "effort syndrome" NEUROCIRCULATORY ASTHENIA

"(the) itch". . . . . . . SCABIES

"itching". . . . . PRURITUS

"jitters". . . . . EXTREME NERVOUSNESS

"jungle rot". . . . . . . FUNGUS INFECTION

"knee cap". . . . . PATELLA (*a small dish*-L)

"knee jerk". . . . . PATELLAR REFLEX

"lice" (head)...... PEDICULOSIS CAPITIS
"liver spots"....... CHLOASMA (from CHLOAZEIN, *to be green*)
"lock jaw"........ TETANUS (from TETAN(OS), *convulsive tension*)
"loss of memory"... AMNESIA
"lumpy jaw"....... ACTINOMYCOSIS
"malignant pustule". ANTHRAX
"malta fever"...... BRUCELLOSIS
"matter".......... PUS; PURULENT DISCHARGE
"measles"......... RUBEOLA
"morning sickness".. VOMITING OF PREGNANCY
"mumps"......... EPIDEMIC PAROTITIS
"nearsightedness"... MYOPIA
"nits"............ LARVAE (EGGS) of PEDICULI (LICE)
"nosebleed"....... EPISTAXIS
"parrot fever"...... PSITTACOSIS (from PSITTAK(OS), *parrot* and OSIS)
"periods"......... MENSTRUATION
"perverted appetite". PICA
"piles"........... HEMORRHOIDS
"pimples"......... ACNE
"pink eye"........ ACUTE CATARRHAL CONJUNCTIVITIS
"pit of the stomach". EPIGASTRIUM
"poison ivy"....... RHUS DERMATITIS
"pregnancy"....... GESTATION
"prickly heat"...... MILIARIA
"pyorrhea"........ PERIODONTITIS
"quinsy (sore throat)"........ PERITONSILLAR ABSCESS
"rabbit fever"...... TULAREMIA
"ringing in the ears"........... TINNITUS-(L)

"roof of mouth". . . .PALATE
"rubbing off of skin" ABRASION
"(the) runs". . . . . . .DIARRHEA
"rupture". . . . . HERNIA
"St. Vitus' dance". . .CHOREA (from CHOREIA, *dance*)
"scar"; "scarred". . . CICATRIX; CICATRIZED
"(the) shakes". . . . .CHILLS; RIGORS
"shaking palsy". . . . PARALYSIS AGITANS
                      (PARKINSON'S DISEASE)
"shin bone". . . . . . .TIBIA
"shiner"; "black
  eye". . . . . ECCHYMOSIS OF EYE
"shingles". . . . . . . .HERPES ZOSTER
"shot"; "hypo". . . . .A HYPODERMIC INJECTION
"sick headache". . . .MIGRAINE (from HEMI, *half* and
                      KRANI(ON), *skull*)
"sleeping sickness". .ENCEPHALITIS LETHARGICA
"small pox". . . . . . .VARIOLA-(L)
"spit"; "spittle". . . .SALIVA; SPUTUM
"(to) spit". . . . . . . (TO) EXPECTORATE
"spitting of blood"
  (from lungs). . . .HEMOPTYSIS
"spotting". . . . . . . .SLIGHT BLOODY VAGINAL DIS-
                      CHARGE
"stitch". . . . . .SUTURE
"stomach pump"
  (use of). . . . . . .GASTRIC LAVAGE
"strawberry mark". .CONGENITAL HEMANGIOMA
"stroke". . . . . CEREBRAL APOPLEXY
"sty". . . . . .HORDEOLUM-(L)
"superfluous hair". . HYPERTRICHOSIS; HIRSUTISM
"sway back". . . . . .LORDOSIS
"sweetbread". . . . . .PANCREAS (from PAN, *all* and
                      CREAS, *flesh*)
"tarry stools". . . . . .MELENA (from MELAN, *black*)

"tennis elbow"......RADIO-HUMERAL BURSITIS
"throw-up" "puke"...VOMIT; EMESIS
"tongue-tie".......ANKYLOGLOSSIA
"treatment".......THERAPY
"trench mouth"....VINCENT'S INFECTION or ULCER-
                    ONECROTIC   GINGIVOSTOMAT-
                    ITIS
"(the) virus"......ANYTHING from a slight INDISPO-
                    SITION to a serious INFECTION
                    caused by a VIRUS
"voice box".......LARYNX
"vomiting of blood".HEMATEMESIS
"wart"...........VERRUCA VULGARIS
"water brash"......REGURGITATION
"wen"............SEBACEOUS CYST
"(the) whites".....LEUCORRHEA
"whooping cough"..PERTUSSIS (from PER, *through*
                    and TUSSIS-L, *cough*)
"wind" (passed
  rectally).......FLATUS-(L)
"wisdom teeth".....THIRD (PERMANENT) MOLARS
"wry neck".......TORTICOLLIS (from TORQUERE-L,
                    to twist and COLL(UM)-L,
                    neck)

COMMON ABBREVIATIONS, THEIR ORIGINS AND MEANINGS

LISTED ARE ABBREVIATIONS and SYMBOLS frequently used in PRESCRIPTION WRITING, MEDICAL RECORDS (office and hospital history charts) and MEDICAL LITERATURE (textbooks and periodicals). All are of Latin origin unless otherwise noted.

āā (ANA) . . . . of each
a.c. (ANTE CIBUM) . before meals
ACTH . . . . adrenocorticotropic hormone
        (from the anterior pituitary)
A.D.A . . . . American Dental Association
ad lib (AD LIBITUM) .at pleasure, or freely
aet (AETATIS) . . . . . at the age of
A/G ratio . . . . albumin globulin ratio
A.M.A . . . . American Medical Association
$A_2 > P_2$ . . . . aortic second heart sound is
        greater than pulmonic second
aq. (AQUA) . . . . water
A.S.H.D . . . . arteriosclerotic heart disease
A.Z. test . . . . Aschheim-Zondek test for preg-
        nancy
B.E . . . . barium enema (x-ray examina-
        tion)
b.i.d. (BIS IN DIE) . . twice daily
B.M . . . . bowel movement
B.M.R . . . . basal metabolic rate
B.P . . . . blood pressure

B.S.P. test........ bromsulphalein test (liver function)

B U N........... blood urea nitrogen

c̄ (CUM)......... with

C............... centigrade

C. (CONGIUS)..... gallon

ca (CIRCA)....... around; about (referring to year)

Ca (CARCINOMA-
    Gr.)........... cancer

C.B.C........... complete blood count

cc.............. cubic centimeter

C.C............. chief complaint

Cf or cf (REFER)... compare

cm.............. centimeter

C.N.S........... central nervous system

CRP............ C—reactive protein

C.V............. cardiovascular

C.V.A........... cerebrovascular accident

D & C.......... dilatation and curettage (uterus)

D.O.A.......... dead on arrival (by ambulance)

E.C.G. or E.K.G... electrocardiogram

E.E.G........... electroencephalogram

e.g. (EXEMPLI
    GRATIA)....... for example

E.N.T........... ear, nose and throat

et al (ET ALII)..... and others (co-authors)

E.S.R........... erythrocyte sedimentation rate

F.............. Fahrenheit

f. or ft. (FAC or
    FIAT)......... make, or let it be made (prescriptions)

F.A.C.P......... Fellow, American College of Physicians

F.A.C.S......... Fellow, American College of Surgeons

F.H. . . . . family history
fluor . . . . fluoroscopy
G.B. . . . . gall bladder
G.C. . . . . gonorrhea (gonococcus infection)
G.I. . . . . gastro-intestinal
Gm. . . . . gram
G.P. . . . . general practitioner
gr. . . . . grain
gtt. (GUTTA) . . . . drops
G.U. . . . . genito-urinary
gyn . . . . gynecology or gynecological
hb. or hgb. . . . . hemoglobin
/H.P.F. . . . . per high power field (microscope)
H.S. or hor. som.
   (HORA SOMNI) . . . at bedtime
ibid (IBIDEM) . . . . . . in the same place
I & D. . . . . incision and drainage
id (IDEM) . . . . the same
i.e. (ID EST) . . . . that is
I.M. . . . . intramuscular
I.Q. . . . . intelligence quotient
I.U. . . . . international units
I.V. . . . . intravenous
J.A.M.A. . . . . Journal of the American Medical Association
k.j. . . . . knee jerk
K.U.B. . . . . kidneys, ureters and bladder
l. or L. . . . . liter
LAB. . . . . clinical laboratory
L.E. . . . . lupus erythematosus
L.L.Q. . . . . left lower quadrant
L.M.D. . . . . local medical doctor
L.U.Q. . . . . left upper quadrant

mEq/L...........milliequivalents per liter
ml...............milliliter
multip.
   (MULTIPARA)....a pregnant woman who has already borne one or more children
N.C.A............neurocirculatory asthenia
N.F..............National Formulary
N.N.R............New and Nonofficial Remedies
NO. (NUMERO)....number
NPN.............non-protein nitrogen (blood)
N.R. or Non.Rep.
   (NON
   REPETATUR)....do not repeat (prescriptions)
N.R.C............National Research Council
O (OCTARIUS).....pint
O.B. or O.B.S......obstetrics
O.D. (OCULUS
   DEXTER).......right eye
O.P.D............out patient department
O.R.............operating room
O.S. (OCULUS
   SINISTER).......left eye
P.A.............pernicious (primary) anemia
para............number of pregnancies (as para 1, 2, 3, 4, etc.)
P.B.I............protein bound iodine
p.c. (POST CIBUM)..after meals
P.H.............past history
pH..............hydrogen ion concentration
P.I..............present illness
P.I.D............pelvic inflammatory disease
Post. or P.M......post-mortem examination or autopsy

primip.
    (PRIMIPARA) . . . . a woman bearing her first child
p.r.n. (PRO
    RE NATA) . . . . whenever necessary
Prog. . . . . prognosis
PSP . . . . phenolsulfonphthalein test (for
                            kidney function)
P.T. . . . . physical therapy
P.X. . . . . physical examination
PZI . . . . protamine zinc insulin
q.d. (QUAQUE DIE) . . every day
q. (2)h. (QUAQUE
    SECUNDA HORA) . . every (2) hours
q.i.d. (QUARTER
    IN DIE) . . . . four times a day
q.n. (QUAQUE
    NOCTE) . . . . every night
q.s. (QUANTUM
    SUFFICIT) . . . . a sufficient quantity
q.v. (QUOD VIDE) . . . which see
r . . . . roentgen unit(s)
® . . . . registered trade-mark status
℞ (RECIPE) . . . . take (prescriptions)
R.B.C. . . . . red blood cells
R.H.D. . . . . rheumatic heart disease
Rh neg. . . . . rhesus factor negative (blood)
R.L.Q. . . . . right lower quadrant
R.U.Q. . . . . right upper quadrant
S. or Sig. (SIGNA) . . . write on label (prescriptions)
S.G.O.T. . . . . serum glutamic oxaloacetic acid
                            TRANSAMINASE TEST
S.O.S. (SI OPUS SIT) . if necessary
sp.gr. . . . . specific gravity
s̄ (SINE) . . . . without
ss (SEMIS) . . . . half

S.S.E. . . . . soap suds enema
stat (STATIM) . . . . . .at once
T & A. . . . . .tonsils and adenoids
Tb or Tbc. . . . . .tuberculosis
t.i.d. (TER IN DIE) . . three times a day
T.P.R. . . . . .temperature, pulse and respiration
U.R.I. . . . . .upper respiratory (tract) infection
U.S.P. . . . . .United States Pharmacopoeia
U.S.P.H.S. . . . . United States Public Health Service
V.D. . . . . .venereal disease
viz. (VIDELICET) . . . namely
W.B.C. . . . . .white blood cells
wt. . . . . weight
♂ . . . . .male
♀ . . . . .female
+ . . . . .plus; positive
− . . . . .minus; negative
± . . . . .positive or negative (not definite)
Q . . . . absent
< . . . . .less than
> . . . . .greater than
° . . . . .degree (s)
mg. % . . . . milligrams per cent
vol. % . . . . volumes per cent
μ . . . . .micron
μg . . . . .microgram
mμ . . . . millimicron

STANDARD NOMENCLATURE

THE NATIONAL CONFERENCE ON NOMENCLATURE OF DISEASE was formed in 1928 for the express purpose of bringing order out of chaos regarding the names of diseases. Many diseases were given various names by different authors. A similar situation prevailed with the names of surgical procedures. This confused state definitely impeded scientific progress.

As a culmination of many years' work by the NATIONAL CONFERENCE, aided by several national scientific organizations and foundations, there appeared in 1933 the first edition of the book, STANDARD NOMENCLATURE OF DISEASES AND OPERATIONS. In 1937, the AMERICAN MEDICAL ASSOCIATION, to keep the profession abreast of the progress of medicine, assumed the responsibility of publishing periodic revisions of this book.

The book classifies all diseases according to TOPOGRAPHY (LOCATION) and ETIOLOGY(CAUSE), assigning a specific code number to each group and subdivision. For example, the DIGESTIVE SYSTEM is designated as code number 6. The fourth organ listed in the digestive system is the STOMACH, so that the number 4 is placed next to 6, making its code number 64. If the lesion (disease) is located in the PYLORUS (code number 5 in list of parts of the stomach), its code number becomes 645. If the etiology of the lesion is a NEW GROWTH (code number -8), then the diagnosis NEW GROWTH OF THE PYLORIC PORTION OF THE STOMACH would be coded 645-8. There are further sub-classifications indicating special symptoms, and other manifestations of disease. The minimum number of digits in any code number is six, and the maximum is twelve.

This standardization of nomenclature, with its systematic scientific schema, has been of inestimable value in furthering medical progress. Its beneficial effects have been reflected in the marked improvement in the accuracy and usefulness of medical records. Medical literature and statistics have thus become so much more valuable to the student of medicine, both young and old, resulting in improved patient care, teaching and research.

The important role of the hospital MEDICAL RECORDS LIBRARIAN in supervising medical records and in seeing that they are properly and thoroughly completed before being filed, cannot be overemphasized.

ANATOMICAL NOMENCLATURE had been in a chaotic state for many years due to the disregard for uniformity in various countries and the myriad of confusing eponyms. In 1895, in Basle, Switzerland, the first attempt at clarification was made by the establishment of the system known as B N A (Basle Nomina Anatomica). All anatomical structures and terms were given standardized Latin names.

To avoid confusion and to facilitate the transition, either the letters B N A or O T (Old Terminology) were placed after each anatomical term. The system, after some necessary revisions, gradually achieved general acceptance. In 1952, anatomists from all countries finally agreed to abide by the B N A regulations in all future editions of textbooks.

Since the beginning of the century, the rapidly expanding knowledge of the etiology, physiology and

pathology of cardiovascular diseases demanded clarification and standardization of its nomenclature. In
1928, the Heart Committee of the New York Tuberculosis and Health Association, Inc., published the first
edition of the book, NOMENCLATURE AND CRITERIA
FOR DIAGNOSIS OF DISEASES OF THE HEART, which was
officially adopted and distributed by the American
Heart Association.

To keep pace with progress, the book has been
periodically revised. In the 1942 edition, in order to
conform with the definition of "disease", as used in the
STANDARD CLASSIFIED NOMENCLATURE OF DISEASE,
each cardiac condition was classified, not only as to
ETIOLOGICAL, ANATOMICAL (structural organic
changes) and PHYSIOLOGICAL aspects, but also as to
FUNCTIONAL CAPACITY.

The latter was classified into four categories according to the ability of the patient to carry on varying degrees of activity, from "no discomfort from ordinary
physical activity" (Class I) to "inability to carry on
any physical activity without discomfort" (Class IV).
Also added was the THERAPEUTIC CLASSIFICATION
(five classes), which prescribed graded physical activity ranging from "no restriction of ordinary physical
activity" (Class A) to "complete bed rest" (Class E).

The same edition also introduced a new "NOMEN-
CLATURE AND CRITERIA FOR THE PATHOLOGICAL
DIAGNOSIS OF CARDIOVASCULAR DISEASES AND ANO-
MALIES," which, by standardizing the terminology of
cardiovascular pathology, filled a long felt need.

CORRECT PRONUNCIATION OF MEDICAL WORDS

T HERE IS GENERAL AGREEMENT on the correct pronunciation of most medical words. However, in certain instances, the correct pronunciation is debatable, even among authorities. Listed below are some of these controversial words, with their correct pronunciation re-spelled phonetically and accented syllables capitalized. Alternative pronunciations are added and those considered less desirable are enclosed in parentheses. Authority for this listing is based on the unanimous or majority opinion of standard English and medical dictionaries, supported by common usage, with few exceptions.

ABDOMEN . . . . ab-DO-men; (AB-do-men)
ADULT . . . . a-DULT; (AD-ult)
ALBUMIN . . . . al-BYOU-min
APNEA . . . . ap-NEE-a
APPARATUS . . . . ap-pa-RAY-tus; (ap-pa-RAT-us)
APPENDICEAL . . . . . ap-pen-DIS-e-al; (ap-pen-di-SEE-al)
AUTOPSY . . . . AW-top-see
BUCCAL . . . . BUCK-al
CAVERNOUS . . . . CAV-er-nous
CEREBRAL . . . . SER-e-bral; (se-REE-bral)
CEREBRUM . . . . SER-e-brum
CHEMOTHERAPY . . . kem-o-THER-a-pee
CITRATES . . . . SIT-rates; (SITE-rates)
COCCI . . . . KOK-seye

COCCYGEAL . . . . .cok-SIJ-e-al
DATA . . . . .DAY-ta; DAT-ta
DIGITALIS . . . . di-gi-TAY-lis
DILATE . . . . di-LATE
DIVERTICULUM . . . . die-ver-TIC-u-lum
DUODENAL . . . . .du-o-DEEN-al
DUODENUM . . . . . . .du-o-DEE-num
DYSPNEA . . . . .disp-NEE-a
EPIPHYSEAL . . . . . . .ep-i-FIZ-e-al
ESOPHAGEAL . . . . . .e-sa-FAJ-e-al: (e-sa-fa-JEE-al)
EXPIRATORY . . . . . . ex-PIE-ra-to-ri
FLACCID . . . . FLAK-sid
FORAMEN . . . . fo-RAY-min
FUNGI . . . . FUN-jeye
GERIATRICS . . . . jerr-ee-AT-ricks
GYNECOLOGY . . . . . .GUY-ne-co-logy; JIN-e-co-logy
HEMOGLOBIN . . . . . .he-mo-GLO-bin
HYPERPNEA . . . . . . .hy-perp-NEE-a
HYPOPHYSEAL . . . . .hy-po-FIZ-e-al
INFANTILE . . . . .IN-fan-tile; (IN-fan-till
INSPIRATORY . . . . . .in-SPY-ra-tor-ri; (IN-spi-ra-to-ri)
IODINE . . . . .EYE-o-dine; EYE-o-din
ISOTOPE . . . . .EYE-so-tope
LARYNGEAL . . . . . . .la-RIN-ge-al
LONGEVITY . . . . . . .lon-JEV-i-ty
MENINGEAL . . . . . . .me-NIN-jee-al
MIGRANE . . . . .MY-grain; MI-grain
OCCULT . . . . .OC-KULT; OCK-ult
ORTHOPNEA . . . . . .or-thop-NEE-a
PHALANGEAL . . . . . .fa-LAN-ge-al
PHARYNGEAL . . . . . .fa-RIN-ge-al
RATIONALE . . . . rash-un-A-lee
RESEARCH . . . . .re-SEARCH; REE-search
RESPIRATORY . . . . . .re-SPY-ra-to-ri; (RES-pi-ra-to-ri)

ROENTGEN........RENT-ghin; RUNT-ghin;
                                (RUNT-yen)
SALICYLATES......SAL-i-cyl-ates; sa-LIS-i-lates
SEQUELA.........se-QUEE-la
STATUS..........STAY-tus; STAT-us
SULFAPYRIDINE....sul-fa-PEER-a-din
SULFONAMIDE.....sul-fon-AM-ide; (sul-FON-amide)
SYNCOPE.........SIN-co-pee
SYNDROME.......SIN-dro-me; SIN-drome
TRICHOMONAS.....tri-KOM-o-nas
UMBILICUS.......um-BIL-i-cus; um-bi-LIE-cus
URETER..........you-REE-ter; YOU-re-ter
VERTEBRAL.......VER-te-bral
VIRUS...........VIE-rus
VISCID..........VIS-id
VITAMIN.........VITE-a-min; (VIT-a-min)

In words such as APHTHOUS, OPHTHALMIC and DIPHTHERIA, the "PH" is preferably pronounced as "F" rather than "P".

The common suffix — ITIS is correctly pronounced -EYE-tis.

In words ending with the suffixes -ITIS -OMA and -OSIS the accent is on next to the last syllable; eg., co-LI-tis; sin-u-SI-tis; sar-CO-ma; a-den-o-ma; neph-RO-sis; scler-o-sis; etc.

In many words ending in -EAL, as DIARRHEAL, GONORRHEAL, LEUCORRHEAL, PERINEAL, PERONEAL, PERITONEAL, etc., the accent is on E (next to the last syllable). Exceptions are certain words (tabulated above) as: APPENDICEAL, COCCYGEAL, EPIPHYSEAL, ESOPHAGEAL, HYPOPHYSEAL, LARYNGEAL, MENINGEAL, PHALANGEAL, and PHARYNGEAL, in which the correct or preferred accent is on the syllable preceding the -EAL. Some of these have alternative pronunciations, as noted in the tabulation.

GENERAL PRACTICE AND
THE SPECIALTIES

THE GENERAL PRACTITIONER, or family physician, has always been, and will continue to be, the backbone of medical practice. Thanks to the commendable program of the American Academy of General Practice in providing frequent refresher courses, the present day general practitioner is kept abreast of all modern advances in medicine. Successful completion of these postgraduate courses and other educational activities are credited towards certification of competency, issued by the Academy.

The SPECIALIST is also here to stay because the tremendous increase in medical knowledge demands prolonged, concentrated study and specialized training to be proficient in any one of the particular fields of medicine. The ever increasing number of medical centers and group clinics throughout the country require well-trained specialists as well as competent general practitioners, the work of each complementing that of the other. Thus, the highest quality of medical care (as well as the most efficient and most economical) may be attained by the combined and cooperative efforts of both of these equally essential, and mutually helpful, groups.

The Advisory Board for Medical Specialties, sponsored by the Council on Medical Education and Hospitals of the American Medical Association, has set up nineteen specialty boards, the purposes of which are: "to establish minimum standards of graduate education and training requirements for physicians representing themselves to the public as being specialists, with certification by the Boards of candidates after they had been able successfully to pass the Boards' (written and oral) examinations".

Following is a list of the AMERICAN BOARDS (with sub-specialties where applicable):

    ANESTHESIOLOGY
    DERMATOLOGY and SYPHILOLOGY
    INTERNAL MEDICINE
        ALLERGY
        CARDIOVASCULAR DISEASE
        GASTROENTEROLOGY
        PULMONARY DISEASES
    NEUROLOGY and PSYCHIATRY
    NEUROLOGICAL SURGERY
    OBSTETRICS and GYNECOLOGY
    OPHTHALMOLOGY
    ORTHOPEDIC SURGERY
    OTOLARYNGOLOGY
    PATHOLOGY
        CLINICAL PATHOLOGY
        PATHOLOGIC ANATOMY
    PEDIATRICS
    PLASTIC SURGERY
    PHYSICAL MEDICINE and REHABILITATION
    PREVENTIVE MEDICINE
        PUBLIC HEALTH
        AVIATION MEDICINE
    PROCTOLOGY
    RADIOLOGY
        ROENTGENOLOGY

DIAGNOSTIC ROENTGENOLOGY

THERAPEUTIC RADIOLOGY

RADIUM THERAPY

SURGERY

THORACIC SURGERY

UROLOGY

The Directory of Medical Specialists, which is revised periodically, lists the names and gives the biographies of all physicians holding certification by the various American Boards. The physicians certified as specialists are also designated as DIPLOMATES of their respective Boards.

Other medical specialties are:

GERIATRICS, from GER(AS), *aged* and IATR(ICS), *healing* or *physician*. Def.: "study of the diagnosis and treatment of diseases of the aged."

ONCOLOGY, from OGKOS, *tumor*, and (O)LOGY, *study of*. Def.: "study of (the diagnosis and treatment of) malignant tumors (cancer)."

In DENTISTRY, the following are recognized as specialties, with certification by their respective boards:

ENDODONTICS or ENDODONTIA, from ENDO, *within* and ODONT, *teeth*. Def.: "treatment of pulpless teeth." (also known as ROOT CANAL THERAPY)

EXODONTIA or EXODONTICS, from EX, *out* and ODONT, *teeth*. Def.: "art and science of extraction of teeth."

ORAL PATHOLOGY

ORAL SURGERY

ORTHODONTICS or ORTHODONTIA, from ORTHO, *straight* and ODONT, *teeth*. Def.: "art and science of straightening teeth, or of treating malocclusion of teeth."

PEDODONTICS or PEDODONTIA, from PED, *child* and

ODONT, *teeth*. Def.: "the special branch of dentistry that treats oral and dental problems in children."

PERIODONTICS or PERIODONTIA, from PERI, *around* and ODONT, *teeth*. Def.: "diagnosis and treatment of diseases of tissues surrounding the teeth."

PROSTHODONTIA or PROSTHODONTICS, from PROSTH (ES), *in addition to* and ODONT, *teeth*. Def.: "study of restoration of teeth by artificial means." (also known as PROSTHETIC DENTISTRY)

SOME MEDICAL TERMS
ANALYZED AND DEFINED

ABERRANT........[ABERRARE-L], *to wander from*
>   Def.: "deviation from the normal form, structure or course."

ACHONDROPLASIA...A, *absence of* + CHONDR(OS), *cartilage* + PLAS(SEIN), *formation*
>   Def.: "a type of dwarfism characterized by very short arms and legs, but with normal sized head and torso, due to a congenital failure in adequate cartilage formation with premature ossification at the ends of the long bones." Its synonym is ACHONDRO-DYSTROPHIA FETALIS.

ACTINOMYCOSIS.... ACTIN (from AKTIS), *ray* + MYC-(ES), *fungus* + OSIS, *condition of being*
>   Def.: "ray fungus infection communicated to humans by affected cattle or hogs."

ACUTE...........[ACUT(US)-L], *sharp*
>   Def.: "sharp or severe; "having a rapid onset, short course or pronounced manifestations." (Opposite to CHRONIC as applied to the stage or course of a disease.)

ADNEXA..........[ADNECTERE, ADNEX(US)-L], *to tie or attach to*
>   Def.: "accessory parts of an organ" e.g., ADNEXA

UTERI are the *uterine tubes* and the *ovaries*.

ALIMENTATION . . . . . [ALIMENT(UM)-L], *food*
Def.: "nourishing with food."

ALLERGY . . . . .ALL(OS), *other* + ERG(ON), *work*
Def.: "altered reaction (sensitivity) to a specific substance."

AMBULATORY . . . . . . [AMBULARE-L], *to walk about*
Def.: "able to walk"; "not confined to bed."

AMYLASE . . . . AMYL(ON), *starch* + ASE, *enzyme*
Def.: "an enzyme that splits (hydrolyzes) starch into sugar."

ANKYLOSIS . . . . AGKYLOS, *crooked* + OSIS.
Def.: "stiffness or fixation of a joint."

ANDROGEN . . . . ANDRO, *man* + GEN, *producing*.
Def.: "male sex hormone."

ANNULAR . . . . [ANULUS-L], *ring*.
Def.: "referring to a ring of tissue around an opening." e.g., ANNULAR CARCINOMA OF THE PYLORUS

ARTEFACT . . . .[ARS, ART(IS)-L], *art* + FACERE-L, *to make*.
Def.: "an artificially produced structure or mark."

ASTHENIA . . . . A, *absence of* + STHEN(OS), *strength*.
Def.: "absence or loss of strength."

ATARAXIA . . . . A, *absence of* + TARAX(IS), *excitement*.
Def.: "absence (or elimination) of excitement"; "state of tranquility." ATARACTIC drugs are also known as TRANQUILIZERS.

ATRESIA. . . . . A, *absence of* + TRES(IS), *per-foration.*

Def.: "closure of normal opening."

BALLISTO-

CARDIOGRAPH. . . . [BALLISTA-L], *military machine for projectiles* + CARDIA, *heart* + GRAPH(EIN), *write.*

Def.: "an instrument that records the movements of the body caused by the impact and recoil of the blood after ejection by the ventricles."

BRACHIAL. . . . . [BRACHI(UM)-L], *arm* + AL, *re-ferring to.*

Def.: "referring to the arm."

BRACHYCEPHALY. . . .BRACHY(S), *short* + CEPHAL(E), *head*

Def.: "shortness of the head."

BRADYCARDIA. . . . . . BRADY(S), *slow* + CARDIA, *heart.*

Def.: "slow rate of the heart beat (pulse)."

BUCCAL. . . . .[BUCC(A)-L], *cheek* + AL, *re-ferring to.*

Def.: "referring to the cheek."

CACHEXIA. . . . . KAK(OS), *bad* + HEX(IS), *state.*

Def.: "state of marked emaciation and weakness."

CATHARSIS. . . . . . . .KATHARSIS, *a cleansing.*

Def.: "purgation."

CAUSALGIA. . . . . . . .KAUS(OS), *heat* + ALGIA, *pain.*

Def.: "a type of burning pain in nerve injury."

CHLOROSIS. . . . . CHLOR(OS), *green* + OSIS.

Def.: "a type of anemia in young women, known as "green sickness" formerly common but hardly ever seen now." The term CHLORO-

PHYL, *the green coloring matter of plants,* has the same derivation.

CHROMOSOME......CHROM(A), *color* + SOMA, *body.*
Def.: "a deeply staining body carrying hereditary factors (genes)"

CHRONIC..........CHRON(OS), *time.*
Def.: "of long duration." (opposite to ACUTE)

CHYLE............CHYL(OS), *juice.*
Def.: "milk-white fat emulsion in lymph, formed in small intestines."

CIRRHOSIS.........KIRRH(OS), *tawny yellow* + OSIS.
Def.: "a progressive inflammatory disease of the liver leading to fibrosis."

CLAUSTROPHOBIA...[CLAUSTR(O)-L], *a confined place* + PHOBIA, *fear.*
Def.: "morbid fear of being in a confined place."

CLINICIAN.........KLIN(E), *bed* +ICIAN, *one who practices at.*
Def.: "a physician who practices at the bedside of a patient as opposed to one who does laboratory or investigative work." The terms CLINIC, POLYCLINIC and CLINICO-PATHOLOGICAL are all derived from the same root.

COLIC............KOLIK(OS), *suffering in the colon.*
Def.: "pertaining to the colon;" "paroxysmal abdominal pain due to colonic spasm."

COLLAGEN.........KOLLA, *glue* + GEN, *producing.*
Def.: "albuminoid substance of connective tissue."

COMA............KOMA, *deep sleep.*
Def.: "unconsciousness."

CRISIS............KRISIS, *turning point.*
Def.: "turning point in a disease."

CRYPTOGENIC......KRYPT(OS), *hidden* + GEN, *caused or produced by.*
   Def.: "of unknown (hidden) cause."

DIAPHORESIS.......DIA, *through* + PHOREO, *carry.*
   Def.: "perspiration."

DIATHESIS.........DIATHESIS, *a placing in order.*
   Def.: "susceptible to a specific disease or condition."

DISTAL........... [DISTARE-L], *to be distant.*
   Def.: "furthest away from a given point." (opposite to PROXIMAL)

DIVERTICULUM.....[DIVERTICULUM-L], *a by-path.*
   Def.: "a pouch arising from a hollow organ."

DYSKINESIA........DYS, *difficult* + KINES(IS), *motion.*
   Def.: "impairment of voluntary motion."

DYSTOCIA......... DYS, *difficult* + TOKOS, *birth.*
   Def.: "difficult labor."

ECTOPIC.......... EC, *out of* + TOP(OS), *place.*
   Def.: "out of place." e.g., ECTOPIC PREGNANCY

EMACIATION.......[EMACIARE-L], *to make lean.*
   Def.: "a wasted condition."

EMBOLUS......... EMBOL(OS), *a plug.*
   Def.: "a plug of (foreign) matter lodged in and obstructing a blood vessel."

ENDOCRINE.......ENDO(N), *within* + CRIN(EIN), *to separate or secrete.*
   Def.: "internally secreting." (referring to the so-called ductless glands.)

ESTROGEN.........[OESTR(US)-L], *heat or female sexual activity* + GEN, *producing.*
   Def.: "female sex hormone."

ETIOLOGY. . . . . AITA, *cause* + LOGOS, *study of.*
   Def.: "the study of the causes of a disease."
EXACERBATION. . . . . [EXACERBARE-L], *to irritate.*
   Def.: "reappearance or increased severity of symptoms." (opposite to REMISSION).
EXUDATE. . . . . EX, *out* + [SUDARE-L], *sweat.*
   Def.: "fluid that has oozed out."
FECES. . . . . .FAEX, *dregs.*
   Def.: "excreta of the bowels."
GONADS. . . . . .GONE, *seed.*
   Def.: "the sex organs." (ovaries and testes).
HEMATOCRIT. . . . . . HEM(AT), *blood* + CRIN(EIN), *to separate.*
   Def.: "a small centrifuge used to separate blood cells." HEMATOCRIT READING is the volume (in per cent of the whole blood volume) of the packed red cells after centrifugation.
HISTOLOGY. . . . . HIST(OS), *tissue* + LOGOS, *study of.*
   Def.: "study (or science) of tissue structure."
HORMONE. . . . . .HORMAIEN, *to excite.*
   Def.: "a specific chemical product of an organ that travels via blood (or other fluid) to affect other remote organs;" "a chemical messenger."
HYPOPHYSIS. . . . . . . HYPO, *below or under* + PHYSIS, *growth.* (literally meaning undergrowth)
   Def.: "the pituitary gland."
INSPIRATION. . . . . . .IN, *in* + SPIRAT(IO), *breathing* + ION, *act of.*
   Def.: "act of breathing in or inhaling."

ISOTOPE.......... ISO(S), *equal* + TOP(OS), *place.*
>Def.: "an element having the same atomic number as another but with a different atomic weight."

JUXTAPOSITION.... [JUXTA-L], *near* + POSITION.
>Def.: "a situation adjacent to another."

KERATIN..........KERAS, *horn.*
>Def.: "the scleroprotein of horny tissue as hair, nails and feathers."

KINETIC.......... KIN(ESIS), *motion* + IC, *pertaining to.*
>Def.: "pertaining to motion."

LESION...........[LAESIO-L], *a hurting.*
>Def.: "a wound, sore, disease or pathological condition.

MENARCHE........MEN, *month* + ARCHE, *beginning.*
>Def.: "the beginning of the menstrual function."

MORBIDITY........[MORBIDUS-L], *disease.*
>Def.: "the quality of disease or of being diseased."

NEPHROTOXIC......NEPHR(OS), *kidney* + TOXIC-(ON), *poison.*
>Def.: "poisonous to the kidney cells."

NEURASTHENIA.....NEUR(ON), *nerve* + A, *absence of* + STHEN(OS), *strength.*
>Def.: "nervous exhustion or neurosis."

OCCULT..........[OCCULTUS-L], *hidden.*
>Def.: "hidden, concealed or not evident." OCCULT BLOOD is blood (in urine, stool, gastric contents, etc.) not visible to the naked eye but detectable only by chemical tests. An OCCULT disease is one the nature of which is not readily determined.

OLIGURIA . . . . OLIG(OS), *scant* + URIA, *urination.*

Def.: "diminution in quantity of urine excreted."

OPTOMETRIST . . . . . .OPT(IK) (OS), *pertaining to eye* + METR(ON), *measurement* + IST.

Def.: "one who tests eyes in order to fit them with glasses, but does not diagnose or treat diseases of the eye." OPTOMETRISTS are not physicians, OPHTHALMOLOGISTS (sometimes called OCULISTS) are physicians with an M.D. degree, specializing in Ophthalmology, thus being the only practitioners qualified by training and license to treat diseases of the eye, either medically or surgically. OPTICIANS are neither physicians nor optometrists but are skilled technicians who supply and fit glasses on the prescription of physicians.

PALLIATION . . . . [PALLIAT(US)-L], *cloaked.*

Def.: "alleviation of symptoms without attempting to cure the disease."

PAROXYSM . . . . .PAROXYSM(US). *irritation.*

Def.: "a sudden attack, spasm, fit or convulsion."

PATHOGNOMONIC . . . PATH(OS), *disease* + GNOMON, *a judge of.*

Def.: "characteristic of a disease."

PENICILLIN . . . .[PENICILLUM-L] *a painter's brush or pencil.*

Def.: "an antibacterial derived from the mold PENICILLIUM NOTATUM." (so named because of the brushlike character of the growth)

PERISTALSIS . . . . PERI, *around* + STALSIS, *con-traction.*

Def.: "rhythmic circular contractions of smooth muscle causing wavelike progression."

PHOTOPHOBIA . . . . . . .PHOTO, *light* + PHOBIA, *fear.*

Def.: "intolerance to, or fear of, light."

POLIOMYELITIS . . . . .POLIO, *gray* + MYEL, *marrow* + ITIS *inflammation of.*

Def.: "a specific viral neurological disease involving the gray matter of spinal cord, commonly referred to by the laiety as "infantile paralysis."

PRENATAL . . . . .PRE, *before* + [NATAL(IS)-L], *born.*

Def.: "before birth."

PROPHYLAXIS . . . . . . PROPHYLAX, *advanced guard.*

Def.: "guarding against (or prevention of) disease."

PROTEIN . . . . PROTEI(OS), *of first rank.*

Def.: "one of the important constituents of food, found chiefly in meat, fish, eggs, milk, cheese, whole cereal grains, peas, beans, etc."

PROTOCOL . . . . .PROTOKOL(ON), *first leaf of a papyrus.*

Def.: "original record of an experiment, autopsy, or clinical examination."

PROXIMAL . . . .[PROXIM(US)-L], *nearest.*

Def.: "nearest to the beginning, central point or median line." (opposite to DISTAL)

PYROGENIC . . . . .PYR, *fire* + GENIC, *producing.*

Def.: "producing fever."

RADIOACTIVE

ISOTOPE........RADIOACTIVE, *emitting radiant energy,* + ISOTOPE.

Def.: "an element rendered radioactive by artificial means." Examples of those that can be so treated are carbon (C), nitrogen (P), sodium (Na), potassium (K), chlorine (Cl), and iodine (I). They are then called *radioactive isotopes* of the respective elements. After being taken into the body, either orally or by injection, these *"tagged"* atoms can be *"traced"* by means of a Geiger counter.

RADIOLOGY........[RADI(US)-L], *radiant energy,* (particularly x-ray, but radium is also included) + (O)LOGY, *science of.*

Def.: "the science of diagnosis by x-ray and treatment by x-ray and radium." ROENTGEN-OLOGY is that branch of medical practice limited to diagnosis and treatment by x-ray. It is so named in honor of ROENTGEN, a German physicist, who discovered the x-ray in 1895.

REMISSION........ [REMISSIO-L], *a sending back.*

Def.: "subsidence of symptoms." (opposite to EXACERBATION).

SAPROPHYTE.......SAPRO, *rotten* + PHYTE, *plant.*

Def.: "an organism living on dead organic matter."

SCHIZOPHRENIA.... SCHIZ, *split* + PHREN, *mind.*

Def.: "dual personality." (one form of dementia precox).

SENESCENCE.......[SENESCERE-L], *to grow old.*
  Def.: "aging."

SIGMOID......... SIGMA, *letter S of the Greek alphabet* + OID, *like.*
  Def.: "a double or S-shaped curve." Because they are thus shaped, several body structures have this adjective applied to them, but it usually refers to the segment of the lower colon leading into the rectum, known as the SIGMOID COLON.

SINUS............ [SINUS-L], *a curve or bay.*
  Def.: "cavity, pocket, or recess."

SOMNAMBULISM....[SOMNUS-L], *sleep* + [AMBULARE-L], *to walk about.*
  Def.: "sleepwalking."

SPASM...........SPASM(OS), *drawing tight.*
  Def.: "a sudden muscular contraction."

SPERMATIC.......[SPERMA-L], *seed.*
  Def.: "pertaining to semen."

SPHINCTER.......SPHIGKTER, *that which binds tight.*
  Def.: "a muscle surrounding and closing an orifice."

STENOSIS......... STEN(OS), *narrowing* + OSIS.
  Def.: "narrowing, constriction or closing of a channel or opening."

STREPTOMYCES.....[STREPTO-L], *curved* + MYC(ES), *fungus.*
  Def.: "an aerobic genus of fungus from which are derived many saprophytic soil species, which are the sources of the following antibiotics":
  STREPTOMYCIN
  CHLORTETRACYCLINE (AUREOMYCIN)

ERYTHROMYCIN (ILOTYCIN)
NEOMYCIN
OXYTETRACYCLINE (TERRAMYCIN)
CHLORAMPHENICOL (CHLOROMYCETIN)

SYNDROME........ SYNDROM(OS), *a running together.*
Def.: "a group of symptoms and signs characteristic of a specific disease or disorder."

SYNERGISM........SYN, *together* + ERG(OS), *work.*
Def.: "the cooperative (and improved) action of
two or more agents or organs." (opposite
to ANTAGONISM).

TACHYPNEA....... TACHY, *fast* + PNEA, *breathing.*
Def.: "rapid breathing."

THROMBOSIS.......THROMBOS, *a lump* + OSIS.
Def.: "formation of a clot of blood within a
blood vessel (or the heart)."

TRANQUILIZER..... [TRANQUILLUS-L], *calm.*
Def.: "a drug that produces a calming effect."

TREMOR.......... [TREMERE-L], *to shake.*
Def.: "a trembling of the voluntary muscles."

VISCERA......... the plural of [VISCUS-L], *an internal organ.*
Def.: "the organs enclosed within the four body
cavities."

VITAMIN..........[VIT(A)-L], *life* + AMINE, *an
ammonia derivative.*
Def.: "certain accessory food factors essential for
normal growth and maintenance of life."
(The term VITAMINE was coined by FUNK
in 1912 in the mistaken belief that all vita-
mins were derived from AMINES. The
original term VITAMINE was changed to
VITAMIN in 1920.)

EXERCISE IN WORD ANALYSIS

A SELECTED LIST of medical terms is presented as an exercise in WORD ANALYSIS. As demonstrated in the preceding chapter, analyze each term by separating it into its component parts. First find and define the *root* or *roots;* then do the same with the *prefix* or *suffix* or both; and finally add together all the elements of the term to arrive at its definition, which, at times may require some modification.

If you are stumped by any term or wish to verify your own definition thereof, you are advised to consult a good medical dictionary. Each trip to the dictionary should be a rewarding adventure, enriching your experience and adding to your storehouse of knowledge. The list of medical terms is as follows:

LIPEMIA	HETEROTOPIC	HISTOPLASMOSIS
CONGENER	POLYNEURITIS	AGRANULOCYTOSIS
ORAD	AMENORRHEA	HYPERCHLORHYDRIA
BILIOUS	PYOSALPINX	HEMICOLECTOMY
EXPIRE	PLEURODYNIA	MACROGLOSSIA
CELIAC	POLYCYSTIC	PSYCHOSOMATIC
BIOLOGY	PERIODONTIST	POLYCHROMATIC
ADENOMA	BRADYPNEA	HEMOCYTOMETER
ODONTOID	TACHYCARDIA	THROMBOCYTOPENIA
POLYPOID	EXODONTIA	PSEUDODIVERTICULUM
HEMATOMA	MELANOSIS	ARTERIOSCLEROSIS
GENERIC	HEMATEMESIS	PYELONEPHRITIS
APLASTIC	ARTHRALGIA	ENCEPHALOGRAM
DIARRHEA	MALNUTRITION	THROMBOPHLEBITIS

HEMOLYSIS	EPIGLOTTIS	METAMORPHOSIS
CHOLEMIA	ANTIBIOTICS	INTRAMUSCULAR
MULTIPARA	CEPHALALGIA	SUPRACLAVICULAR
UREMIA	HYPERTROPHY	HYPERSENSITIVITY
EXCISION	ENDOCARDITIS	DERMOGRAPHIA
MICROBE	PHLEBOTOMY	OSTEOMYELITIS
BIOPSY	STOMATITIS	PYOPNEUMOTHORAX
MASTITIS	CRANIOTOMY	GASTROENTEROSTOMY
MUCOID	OSTEOPATHY	ILEOCOLOSTOMY
OSTEOMA	MENINGITIS	ERYTHROCYTHEMIA
CUTANEOUS	ANTIPYRETIC	THORACOPLASTY
LEUCOCYTE	PROTOPLASM	CHOLELITHIASIS
MYELOMA	RHINOPLASTY	HEMATOGENOUS
TROPHIC	PERICARDITIS	SUBDIAPHRAGMATIC
PARALYSIS	HEMATOLOGY	CEREBROSPINAL
MICROTOME	CHOLECYSTITIS	OPHTHALMOLOGIST
PNEUMONIA	HYDROTHORAX	HYPERTHYROIDISM
DYSENTERY	PYLORECTOMY	GASTROPTOSIS
UROGRAPHY	PROCTOSCOPY	LYMPHADENITIS
PHONETICS	PARATHYROID	GALACTOSURIA
CIRCUMORAL	EDENTULOUS	ENDOMETRIOSIS
CHYLURIA	HEPATOMEGALY	COCCYGODYNIA
OTALGIA	DICEPHALOUS	DERMATOPHYTOSIS
ODONTALGIA	SPLENECTOMY	ENDOCRINOLOGY
PHLEBOLITH	TRACHEOTOMY	EXPECTORATION

EXERCISE IN WORD BUILDING

To SUPPLEMENT the preceding exercise in word analysis, you may now practice WORD BUILDING. For example, from the root CYT(E), *cell,* the following terms can be constructed: CYTOBLAST, CYTOPLASM, LEUCOCYTE, CYTOLYSIS, ERYTHROCYTE, LYMPHOCYTE, CYTOGENESIS, PHAGOCYTE, etc. As an exercise, take the common roots HEM(O)(AT), *blood;* GASTR(O), *stomach;* and NEPHR(O), *kidney;* and see how many terms you can form by combining each root with another root, a prefix or suffix, or both.

Similarly, by adding various roots to the prefix MACRO-, *large,* we can produce the following terms: MACROCYTE, MACROGLOSSIA, MACROSCOPIC, MACRO-CEPHALY, MACROPHAGE, MACROMASTIA, etc. Now, see how many terms you can build with the following common prefixes and suffixes by combining each one with various roots: PERI-, *around;* POST-, *after;* PSEUDO-, *false;* -ITIS, *inflammation of;* -ASIS *or* -OSIS, *condition of being;* -GRAPH(Y), *writing* or *description;* -(O)-scopy, *inspection* or *looking into;* and -OMA, *tumor of.*

CONCLUSION

LEARNING MEDICAL TERMINOLOGY, with the resultant acquisition of a rich medical vocabulary, is not as difficult as may appear when one is first confronted by seemingly unpronouncable and unintelligible medical terms.

The first step is to memorize the important and commonly used *roots, prefixes, suffixes* and *combining terms*. Then, after learning a few *principles of word construction,* practice word analysis, constantly referring to a good *medical dictionary,* until the meanings of the terms become as familiar as are common English words.

By this time it should be obvious to the reader that this book is not intended to replace the medical dictionary. On the contrary, constant use of the latter is again strongly advocated and, in fact, is considered essential if one wishes to become proficient in the understanding and correct use of medical terms.

This short treatise is merely a guide to a vast, almost limitless, field of knowledge. Its purpose is to help the student overcome his first, and sometimes persistent, fear of medical terms by showing him how to analyze them himself and with the aid of the medical dictionary.

While thus gradually acquiring an extensive medical vocabulary, the student will be enjoying the absorbing pastime of word analysis as well as learning many

101

interesting facets of the history of medicine, from ancient to modern times.

It is sincerely hoped that this book will succeed in achieving the objective expressed in its title and, besides, be provocative in stimulating the reader to delve more deeply into the subject.

Of the many authoritative text books and reference works consulted by the author in the preparation of this book, the following are particularly recommended to the serious student for supplementary reading.

MEDICAL GREEK AND LATIN AT A GLANCE, by Walter R. Agard
  (Paul B. Hoeber, New York, 1947)

ORIGIN OF MEDICAL TERMS, by H. Alan Skinner
  (Williams & Wilkins Co., Baltimore, 1949)

MEDICAL ETYMOLOGY, by O. H. Perry Pepper
  (W. B. Saunders Co., Philadelphia, 1949)

MEDICAL TERMINOLOGY MADE EASY, by J. C. Harned
  (Physicians' Record Co., Chicago, 1951)

A SOURCE OF MEDICAL TERMS, by Edmund C. Jaeger
  (Charles C Thomas, Springfield, Ill., 1953)

MEDICAL TERMS, THEIR ORIGIN AND CONSTRUCTION, by F. Roberts
  (Charles C Thomas, Springfield, Ill., 1955)

Finally, constant use of a good medical dictionary is again strongly recommended. Of the many frequently referred to by the author, the following have been found most useful:

BLAKISTON'S NEW GOULD MEDICAL DICTIONARY
  Second edition
  (McGraw-Hill Book Co., New York, 1956)

Dorland's American Illustrated Medical Dictionary
  Twenty-third edition
    (W. B. Saunders Co., Philadelphia, 1957)
Stedman's Medical Dictionary
  Nineteenth edition
    (The Williams and Wilkins Co., Baltimore, 1957)